The Amazing Liver & Gallbladder Flush

Also by Andreas Moritz

• • •

Timeless Secrets of Health and Rejuvenation

Lifting the Veil of Duality

Cancer Is Not a Disease (New)

It's Time to Come Alive

Simple Steps to Total Health

Heart Disease No More!

Diabetes—No More!

Ending the AIDS Myth

Heal Yourself With Sunlight!

Hear the Whispers, Live Your Dream (July 2007)

Sacred Santémony

Ener-Chi Art

All of the above are available at **www.ener-chi.com,**
www.amazon.com, and other online or physical bookstores.

The Amazing Liver & Gallbladder Flush

A Powerful Do-It-Yourself Tool
to Optimize Your Health and Well-Being

Andreas Moritz

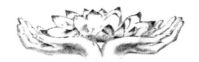

Your Health is in Your Hands

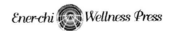

Ener-chi Wellness Press

For Reasons of Legality

The author of this book, Andreas Moritz, does not advocate the use of any particular form of health care but believes that the facts, figures, and knowledge presented herein should be available to every person concerned with improving his or her state of health. Although the author has attempted to give a profound understanding of the topics discussed and to ensure accuracy and completeness of any information that originates from any other source than his own, he and the publisher assume no responsibility for errors, inaccuracies, omissions, or any inconsistency herein. Any slights of people or organizations are unintentional. This book is not intended to replace the advice and treatment of a physician who specializes in the treatment of diseases. Any use of the information set forth herein is entirely at the reader's discretion. The author and publisher are not responsible for any adverse effects or consequences resulting from the use of any of the preparations or procedures described in this book. The statements made herein are for educational and theoretical purposes only and are mainly based on Andreas Moritz's own opinion and theories. You should always consult with a health care practitioner before taking any dietary, nutritional, herbal, or homeopathic supplement, or before beginning or stopping any therapy. The author is not intending to provide any medical advice or offer a substitute thereof, and makes no warranty whatsoever, whether expressed or implied, with respect to any product, device, or therapy. Except as otherwise noted, no statement in this book has been reviewed or approved by the United States Food and Drug Administration or the Federal Trade Commission. Readers should use their own judgment or consult a holistic medical expert or their personal physicians for specific applications to their individual problems.

ISBN: 0-9765715-0-1

Published by Ener-Chi Wellness Press—Ener-chi.com, USA
First edition, *The Amazing Liver Cleanse,* 1998
Second edition, *The Amazing Liver Cleanse,* 1999 (revised)
Third edition, *The Amazing Liver Cleanse,* USA, 2002 (revised)
Fourth edition, *The Amazing Liver and Gallbladder Flush,* USA, 2005 (extended and revised)
Fifth edition, *The Amazing Liver and Gallbladder Flush,* USA, Feb. 2007 (improved and reedited)
Cover Design/Artwork (Ener-chi Art for the Liver): By Andreas Moritz

Clinical success is the final test.
This book is transforming our current medical model.
Be prepared to be WELL.

"This is more than a book—this is a powerful self-healing tool. At a time when we have given up on our body's own innate wisdom, Andreas Moritz offers a simple, self-directed remedy allowing for one's own self-empowered healing. It is simple, inexpensive, and easy to perform. The healing that occurred for my patients and myself has been life altering."
—**Gene L. Pascucci, BS, DDS** (dentist, metaphysician and mystic living in Reno, Nevada)

"I was intrigued to learn about the liver flush from a friend, although I put off doing it for a good few months. Having suffered from severe health problems for several years, I eventually took the plunge, but not really expecting any great results. Much to my amazement, the next day I excreted about six hundred gallstones of varying sizes and colors, and the relief was instantaneous. I was calmer, felt much less irritable, and had greater clarity of thought. I have now completed five flushes and am nearly back to normal functioning. Whilst I have used other treatment modalities in addition to this cleansing technique, I consider that the liver flush has had a major impact upon my recovery. I shall certainly be adding it to my health maintenance program for the rest of my life."
—**Dr. Diane Phillips, MB, BS, BSc** (UK)

Dedication

*To all those who wish to take responsibility
for their own health and who care about
the health and well-being of their
fellow human beings*

Table of Contents:

INTRODUCTION

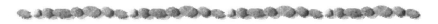

Many people believe that gallstones can be found only in the gallbladder. This is a commonly made yet false assumption. Most gallstones are actually formed in the liver, and comparatively few occur in the gallbladder. You can easily verify this assessment by giving yourself a liver flush. It matters little whether you are a layperson, a medical doctor, a scientist, or someone whose gallbladder was removed and, therefore, is believed to be stone free. The results of the liver flush[1] speak for themselves. No amount of scientific proof or medical explanation can make such a cleanse any more valuable than it already is. Once you see hundreds of green, beige-colored, brown, or black gallstones floating in the toilet bowl during your first liver flush, you will intuitively know that you are on to something extremely important in your life. To satisfy your possibly curious mind, you may decide to take the expelled stones to a laboratory for chemical analysis or ask your doctor what she thinks about all that. Your doctor may either support you in your initiative to heal yourself, tell you this is just ridiculous, or warn you against it. However, what is most significant in this experience is that you have taken active responsibility for your own health, perhaps for the first time in your life.

Not everyone is as fortunate as you are. An estimated 20 percent of the world's population will develop gallstones in their *gallbladder* at some stage in their lives; many of them will opt for surgical removal of this important organ. This statistical figure does not account, though, for the many more people who will develop gallstones (or already have them) in their *liver*. During some thirty years of practicing natural medicine and dealing with thousands of people suffering from all types of chronic diseases, I can attest to the fact that each one of them, without exception, has

---

[1] When I refer to the *liver flush*, it includes flushing of the gallbladder as well.

had considerable quantities of gallstones in his or her liver. Surprisingly, only relatively few of them reported to have had a history of gallstones in their gallbladder. Gallstones in the liver are, as you will understand from reading this book, the main impediment to acquiring and maintaining good health, youthfulness, and vitality. Gallstones in the liver are, indeed, one of the major reasons people become ill and have difficulty recuperating from illness.

The failure to recognize and accept the incidence of gallstone formation in the liver as an extremely common phenomenon may very well be the most unfortunate oversight that has ever been made in the field of medicine, both orthodox and holistic.

Relying so heavily on blood tests for diagnostic purposes, as conventional medicine does, may actually be a great disadvantage with regard to assessing liver health. Most people who have a physical complaint of one kind or another may show to have perfectly normal liver enzyme levels in the blood, despite suffering from liver congestion. Liver congestion is among the leading health problems, yet conventional medicine rarely refers to it, nor do doctors have a reliable way to detect and diagnose such a condition. Liver enzyme levels in the blood become elevated only when there is advanced liver cell destruction, as is the case, for example, in hepatitis or liver inflammation. Liver cells contain large amounts of enzymes. Once a certain number of liver cells are ruptured, their enzymes will start showing up in the blood. When detected through a blood test, this increased count of liver enzymes indicates abnormal liver functions. In such an event, however, the damage has already occurred. It takes many years of chronic liver congestion before liver damage becomes apparent.

Standard clinical tests almost never reveal the occurrence of gallstones in the liver. In fact, most doctors don't even know they grow there. Only some of the most advanced research universities, such as the prestigious Johns Hopkins University, describe and illustrate these liver stones in their literature or on their web sites. They refer to them as "intrahepatic gallstones."[2]

---

[2] On the Internet, search for *Johns Hopkins Medical Institutions.* Then locate *Digestive Disease Library,* click on *Biliary Tract,* choose *Cholangiocarcinoma,*

By understanding how gallstones in the liver contribute to the occurrence or deterioration of nearly every kind of illness, and by taking the simple steps to remove them, you will put yourself in charge of restoring your own health and vitality, permanently. The implications of applying the liver flush for yourself—or, if you are a health practitioner, for your patients—are immensely rewarding. To have a clean liver equals having a new lease on life.

The liver has direct control over the growth and functioning of every cell in the body. Any kind of malfunction, deficiency, or abnormal growth pattern of the cell is largely due to poor liver performance. Even when it has lost up to 60 percent of its original efficiency, the liver's extraordinary design and resourcefulness may allow it to perform "properly," as indicated by normal blood values. As misleading as this may be to the patient and his doctor, the origin of most diseases can easily be traced to the liver. The first chapter of this book is dedicated to this vitally important connection.

All diseases or symptoms of ill health are caused by an obstruction of some sort. For example, a blood capillary that is blocked can no longer deliver vital oxygen and nutrients to a group of cells it is in charge of supplying. To survive, these cells will need to enforce specific survival measures. Of course, many of the afflicted cells will not live through the "famine" and will simply die off. Yet other, more resilient cells will adjust to this adverse situation through the process of cell mutation and learn to utilize trapped metabolic waste products, such as lactic acid, to cover their energy needs. These cells may be compared to a man in the desert who, for lack of water, relies on drinking his own urine in order to live a little longer than he would otherwise. Cell mutation leading to cancer is only the body's final attempt to help prevent its immediate demise through septic poisoning and a collapsing organ structure. Although common practice, it is far-fetched to call the body's normal response to the accumulation of toxic waste matter and decomposing cell material a disease. Unfortunately, ignorance of the body's true nature has caused many to believe that this

go to bottom of page, and click on *Next Section.* Repeat more times; then scroll down to the last illustration on that page.

survival mechanism is an "autoimmune disease." The word "autoimmune" suggests that the body attempts to attack itself and practically tries to commit suicide. Nothing could be further from the truth. Cancerous tumors result from major congestion in the connective tissues, blood vessel walls, and lymphatic ducts, all of which prevent healthy cells from receiving enough oxygen and other vital nutrients.[3]

Other, more apparent obstructions can disrupt your well-being just as much. A constipated large intestine prevents the body from eliminating the waste products contained in feces. The holding back of fecal matter in the lower parts of the intestinal tract leads to a toxic environment in the colon and, if the situation is not resolved, in the entire body.

Kidney infection and kidney failure may occur in response to the accumulation of calcified stones or deposits of kidney grease, thereby obstructing the flow of urine in the kidneys or urinary bladder. The buildup of such mineral deposits in the urinary system can lead to fluid retention, weight gain, and dozens of disease symptoms.

If acidic, toxic waste matter builds up in the chest and lungs, the body responds with mucus secretions to trap these noxious substances. As a result, the air passages of your lungs become congested, and you literally run out of breath. If your body is already highly toxic and congested, you may even develop a lung infection. Lung infections occur to help destroy and remove any damaged, weak lung cells that otherwise would start rotting or have already been decomposed (pus formation). Lung congestion prevents the natural removal of damaged or weak cells. If the congestion is not cleared up through natural means, or if it increases further through poor dietary habits, the pus will be trapped in the lung tissue. Naturally, destructive bacteria will increasingly populate the scene to assist the body in its desperate effort to clear up this congested area, which comprises decomposing cells and other waste products. Doctors call this survival mechanism "staph infection," or pneumonia.

---

[3] For a complete understanding of what cancer actually is and what causes it, see the author's book *Cancer Is Not a Disease—It's a Survival Mechanism.*

Poor hearing and ear infections may result if sticky mucus filled with toxins and/or dead or live bacteria enter the ducts that run from your throat to your ears (Eustachian tubes). Likewise, thickening of the blood caused by highly acid-forming foods or beverages may restrict its flow through the capillaries and arteries, and thereby lead to numerous conditions, ranging from simple skin irritation to arthritis or high blood pressure, even heart attack and stroke.

These or similar obstructions in the body are directly or indirectly linked to restricted liver performance—in particular, to an impasse caused by gallstones in the liver and gallbladder. The presence of chunks of hardened bile and other trapped organic or inorganic substances in these organs greatly interferes with such vital processes as the digestion of food, elimination of waste, and detoxification of harmful substances in the blood. By decongesting the liver bile ducts and the gallbladder, the body's 60 to 100 trillion cells will be able to "breathe" more oxygen, receive sufficient amounts of nutrients, efficiently eliminate their metabolic waste products, and maintain perfect communication links with the nervous system, endocrine system, and all other parts of the body.

Almost every patient suffering a chronic illness has excessive amounts of gallstones in the liver. A doctor can easily confirm this by having her chronically ill patient do a liver flush. It is apparent that unless a specific liver disease is found, this vital organ is rarely considered a "culprit" for other diseases. The majority of gallstones in the liver consist of the same "harmless" constituents as are found in liquid bile, with cholesterol being the main ingredient. A number of stones consist of fatty acids and other organic material that has ended up in the bile ducts. The fact that the majority of these stones are just congealed clumps of bile or organic matter makes them practically "invisible" to x-rays, ultrasonic technologies, and *computerized tomography* (CT).

The situation is different with regard to the gallbladder, where up to about 20 percent of all stones can be made up entirely of minerals, predominantly calcium salts and bile pigments. Whereas diagnostic tests can easily detect these hardened, relatively large stones in the gallbladder, they tend to miss the softer, noncalcified stones in the liver. Only when excessive amounts of cholesterol-based stones (85–95 percent cholesterol), or other clumps of fat, block the bile ducts of the liver may an ultrasound test reveal what is generally referred to as "fatty liver." In such a case, the ultrasound pictures reveal a liver that is almost completely white (instead of black). A fatty liver can gather up to 20,000 stones before it succumbs to suffocation and ceases to function.

If you had a fatty liver and went to the doctor, she would tell you that you had excessive fatty tissue in your liver. It is less likely, though, that she would tell you that you had *intrahepatic gallstones* (stones obstructing the liver's bile ducts). As mentioned before, most of the smaller stones in the liver are not detectable through ultrasound or CT scans. Nevertheless, careful analysis of diagnostic images by specialists would show whether some of the smaller bile ducts in the liver were dilated because of obstruction. A dilation of bile ducts caused by larger and denser stones or by clusters of stones may be detected more readily through *magnetic resonance imaging* (MRI). However, unless there is an indication of major liver trouble, doctors rarely check for such intrahepatic stones. Unfortunately, although the liver is one of the most important organs in the body, its disorders are also underdiagnosed all too often.

Even if the early stages of a fatty liver or gallstone formation in the bile ducts were easily recognized and diagnosed, today's medical facilities offer no treatments to relieve this vital organ of the heavy burden it has to carry.

Most people in the developed world have accumulated hundreds and, in many cases, thousands of hardened bile and fat deposits in the liver. These stones continuously block the liver's bile ducts, which greatly stresses this vital organ and the rest of the body. In view of the adverse effect these stones have on liver performance as a whole, their composition is quite irrelevant. Whether your doctor or you consider them conventional mineral-based gallstones, fat deposits, or clots of hardened bile, the net result is that they prevent the necessary amounts of bile from reaching the intestines. The important question is how such a simple thing as obstructed bile flow can cause such complex diseases as congestive heart failure, diabetes, and cancer.

Liver bile is a bitter, alkaline fluid of a yellow, brown, or green color. It has multiple functions. Each one of these profoundly influences the health of every organ and system in the body. Apart from assisting with the digestion of fat, calcium, and protein foods, bile is needed to maintain normal fat levels in the blood, remove toxins from the liver, help maintain proper acid/alkaline balance in the intestinal tract, and keep the colon from breeding harmful microbes. To maintain a strong and healthy digestive system and feed body cells the right amount of nutrients, the liver has to produce 1–1.5 quarts of bile per day. Anything less than that is bound to cause problems with the digestion of food, elimination of waste, and the body's continual detoxification of the blood. Many people produce just about a cupful of bile or less per day. As will be shown in this book, almost all health problems are a direct or indirect consequence of reduced bile availability.

People with chronic illnesses often have several thousand gallstones congesting the bile ducts of the liver. Some stones may have also grown in the gallbladder. By removing these stones from these organs through a series of liver flushes and maintaining a balanced diet and lifestyle, the liver and gallbladder can restore their original efficiency, and most symptoms of discomfort or disease in the body can start subsiding. You may find that any persistent allergies will lessen or disappear. Back pain will dissipate, while energy and well-being will improve. Ridding the liver bile ducts of gallstones is one of the most important and powerful procedures you can apply to improve and regain your health.

In this book, you will learn how to remove painlessly up to several hundred gallstones at a time. The size of the stones ranges from that of a pinhead to a small walnut, and in some rare cases a golf ball. The actual liver flush takes place within a period of less than fourteen hours and can be taken conveniently over a weekend at home. Chapter 1 explains in detail why the presence of gallstones in the bile ducts, both inside and outside the liver, can be considered the greatest health risk and cause of almost every major or minor illness. In Chapter 2, you will be able to identify the signs, marks, and symptoms that indicate the presence of stones in your liver or gallbladder. Other chapters deal with the possible causes of gallstones and what you can do to prevent new ones from occurring. In Chapter 4, you will learn the actual procedure to rid your body of gallstones. Chapter 6, "What Can I Expect from the

Liver and Gallbladder Flush?" covers some of the possible health benefits of this profound self-help program. In addition, you will find out what others have to say about their experiences with the liver flush. The frequently asked questions section, Chapter 8, deals with many queries you may have about the flush. To reap the maximum benefit from this procedure, I strongly encourage you to read the entire book before starting with the actual liver flush.

The picture shown on the cover of the book is part of a series of energized oil paintings, known as Ener-Chi Art, that I created to restore the life force energy (Chi) in all the organs and systems of the body. The photographic print of this particular picture helps to restore Chi-flow in the liver and gallbladder. (Unfortunately, digital prints such as the one shown on the book cover do not have this effect; to order photo prints, see *Other Books, Products, and Services by the Author.*) Viewing this picture for at least thirty seconds and preferably longer—before, during, and after the flush—energizes these two organs and may thereby assist you in the process of cleansing and rejuvenating them. The picture, though, is not necessary to achieve excellent results.

I wish you the greatest success on your journey to achieving a perpetual state of health, happiness, and vitality!

Chapter 1

Gallstones in the Liver: A Major Health Risk

Think of the liver as a large city with thousands of houses and streets. There are underground pipes for delivering water, oil, and gas. Sewage systems and garbage trucks remove the city's waste products. Power lines deliver energy to the homes and businesses. Factories, transport systems, communication networks, and stores meet the daily requirements of the residents. The organization of city life is such that it can provide all that it needs for the continued existence of the population. But if a major strike, a power outage, a devastating earthquake, or a major act of terrorism, such as the one we witnessed in New York City on September 11, 2001, suddenly paralyzes city life, the population will begin to suffer serious shortcomings in all these vital sectors.

Like a city's infrastructure, the liver has hundreds of different functions and is connected with every part of the body. Every moment of the day, it is involved in manufacturing, processing, and supplying vast amounts of nutrients. These nutrients feed the 60 to 100 trillion inhabitants (cells) of the body. Each cell is, in itself, a microscopic city of immense complexity, with billions of chemical reactions per second. To sustain the incredibly diverse activities of all the cells of the body without disruption, the liver must supply them with a constant stream of nutrients, enzymes, and hormones. With its intricate labyrinth of veins, ducts, and specialized cells, the liver needs to be completely unobstructed in order to maintain a problem-free production line and frictionless distribution system throughout the body.

The liver is the main organ responsible for distributing and maintaining the body's "fuel" supply. Furthermore, its activities include the breaking down of complex chemicals and the synthesis of protein molecules. The liver acts as a cleansing device; it also deactivates hormones, alcohol, and medicinal drugs. Its task is to modify these biologically active substances so that they lose their potentially harmful effects—a process known as detoxification. Specialized cells in the liver's blood vessels (Kupffer cells) mop up harmful elements and infectious organisms reaching the liver from the gut. The liver excretes the waste materials resulting from these actions via its bile duct network.

A healthy liver receives and filters 3 pints of blood per minute and produces 1 to 1.5 quarts of bile every day. This ensures that all the activities in the liver and in the rest of the body run smoothly and efficiently. Obstructive gallstones greatly undermine the liver's ability to detoxify any externally supplied and internally generated harmful substances in the blood. These stones also prevent the liver from delivering the proper amounts of nutrients and energy to the right places in the body at the right time. This upsets the delicate balance in the body, known as "homeostasis," thus leading to disruption of its systems and undue stress on its organs.

A clear example for such a disturbed balance is an increased concentration of the endocrine hormones *estrogen* and *aldosterone* in the blood. These hormones, produced in both men and women, are responsible for the correct amount of salt and water retention. When stones congest the gallbladder and the liver's bile ducts, these hormones may not be broken down and detoxified sufficiently. Hence, their concentration in the blood rises to abnormal levels, causing tissue swelling and water retention. Most oncologists consider elevated estrogen levels to be the leading cause of breast cancer among women. In men, high levels of this hormone can lead to excessive development of breast tissue and weight gain.

Over 60 percent of the American population is overweight or obese. Men, women, and children in this condition suffer mainly from fluid retention (with relatively minor fat accumulation). The retained fluids help trap and neutralize noxious substances that the liver can no longer remove from the body. This helps the overweight or obese person to survive a major, possibly fatal, toxicity crisis such as a heart attack, septic poisoning, or massive infection. The side effect of fluid retention in the tissues, however, is that it causes these toxins and other harmful waste matter (metabolic waste and dead cell material) to accumulate in various parts of the body and further congest the pathways of circulation and elimination. Wherever in the body the storage capacity for toxins and waste is exceeded, symptoms of illness begin to occur.

Cleansing the liver and gallbladder from all accumulated stones (see **Figures 1a and 1b**) helps to restore homeostasis, balances weight, and sets the precondition for the body to heal itself. The liver flush is also one of the best precautionary measures you can take to protect yourself against nearly every kind of illness, known or unknown.

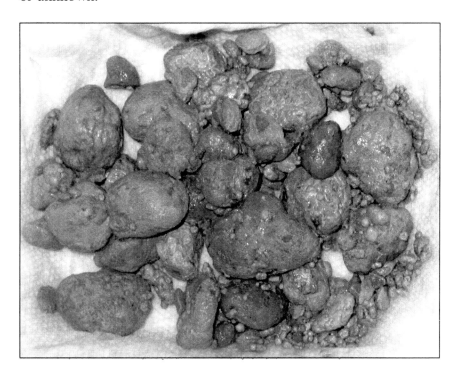

Figure 1a: Flushed-out gallstones

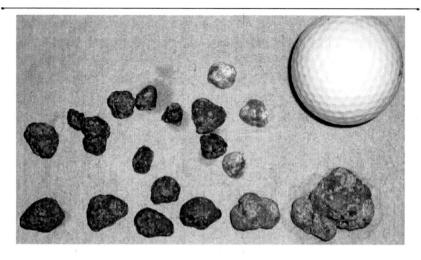

Figures 1b: Flushed-out gallstones

If you suffer any of the following symptoms, or similar conditions, you most likely have numerous gallstones in your liver and gallbladder:

➢ Low appetite
➢ Food cravings
➢ Digestive disorders
➢ Diarrhea
➢ Constipation
➢ Clay-colored stool
➢ Hernia
➢ Flatulence
➢ Hemorrhoids
➢ Dull pain on the right side
➢ Difficulty breathing
➢ Liver cirrhosis
➢ Hepatitis
➢ Most infections
➢ High cholesterol
➢ Pancreatitis
➢ Heart disease
➢ Brain disorders
➢ Duodenal ulcers
➢ Nausea and vomiting
➢ A "bilious" or angry personality
➢ Depression
➢ Impotence
➢ Other sexual problems
➢ Prostate diseases
➢ Urinary problems
➢ Hormonal imbalances
➢ Menstrual and menopausal disorders
➢ Problems with vision
➢ Puffy eyes
➢ Any skin disorder
➢ Liver spots, especially those on the back of the hands and facial area

➢ Dizziness and fainting spells
➢ Loss of muscle tone
➢ Excessive weight or wasting
➢ Strong shoulder and back pain
➢ Pain at the top of a shoulder blade and/or between the shoulder blades
➢ Dark color under the eyes
➢ Morbid complexion
➢ Tongue that is glossy or coated in white or yellow
➢ Scoliosis
➢ Gout
➢ Frozen shoulder
➢ Stiff neck
➢ Asthma
➢ Headaches and migraines
➢ Tooth and gum problems
➢ Yellowness of the eyes and skin

➢ Sciatica
➢ Numbness and paralysis of the legs
➢ Joint diseases
➢ Knee problems
➢ Osteoporosis
➢ Obesity
➢ Chronic fatigue
➢ Kidney diseases
➢ Cancer
➢ Multiple Sclerosis and fibromayalgia
➢ Alzheimer's disease
➢ Cold extremities
➢ Excessive heat and perspiration in the upper part of the body
➢ Very greasy hair and hair loss
➢ Cuts or wounds that keep bleeding and don't want to heal
➢ Difficulty sleeping, insomnia
➢ Nightmares
➢ Stiffness of joints and muscles
➢ Hot and cold flashes

The Importance of Bile

As already mentioned, one of the liver's most important functions is to produce bile, about 1 to 1.5 quarts per day. Liver bile is a viscous, yellow, brown, or green fluid that is alkaline (versus acidic) and has a bitter taste. Without sufficient bile, most commonly eaten foods remain undigested or partially digested. For example, to enable the small intestines to digest and absorb fat and calcium from the food you eat, the food must first combine with bile. When fat is not absorbed properly, it indicates that bile secretion is insufficient. The undigested fat remains in the intestinal tract. When undigested fat reaches the colon along with other waste products, bacteria break down some of the fat into fatty acids or excrete it with the stool. Since fat is lighter than water, having fat in the stool may cause it to float. When fat is not absorbed, calcium is not absorbed either, leaving the blood in a deficit. The blood subsequently takes its extra calcium from the bones. Most bone density problems (osteoporosis) actually arise from insufficient bile secretion and poor digestion of fats, rather than from not consuming enough calcium. Few medical practitioners are aware of this fact and, hence, merely prescribe calcium supplements to their patients.

Apart from breaking down the fats in our food, bile also removes toxins from the liver. One of the lesser known but extremely important functions of bile is to deacidify and cleanse the intestines.

When gallstones in the liver or gallbladder have critically impeded bile flow, the color of the stool may be tan, orange-yellow, or pale as in clay, instead of the normal greenish-brown.

Gallstones are a direct product of an unhealthy diet and lifestyle. If gallstones are still present in the liver even after all other disease-causing factors are eliminated, they pose a considerable health risk and may lead to illness and premature aging. For this reason, the subject of gallstones has been included here as a major risk factor or cause of disease. The following sections describe some of the main consequences of gallstones in the liver on the different organs and systems in the body. When these stones are removed, the body as a whole can resume its normal, healthy activities.

Disorders of the Digestive System

The alimentary tract of the digestive system maintains the following four main activities: *ingestion, digestion, absorption,* and *elimination.* The alimentary canal begins in the mouth; leads through the thorax, abdomen, and pelvic region; and ends at the anus (see **Figure 2**). When you eat a meal, a series of digestive processes begin to take place. These can be divided into the *mechanical breakdown* of food through mastication (chewing) and the *chemical breakdown* of food through enzymes. These enzymes are present in the secretions produced by various glands of the digestive system.

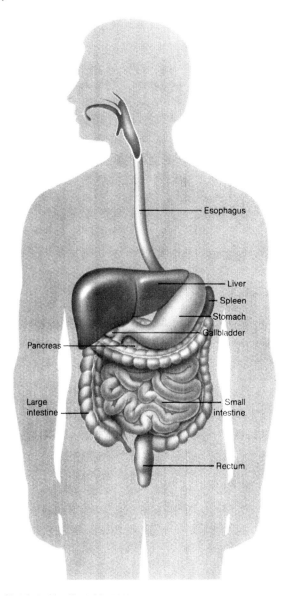

Figure 2: The digestive system

Enzymes are minute chemical substances composed of proteins that cause or speed up chemical changes in other substances without themselves being changed. Digestive enzymes are contained in the saliva of the salivary glands of the mouth, the gastric juice in the stomach, the intestinal juice in the small intestine, the pancreatic juice in the pancreas, and the bile in the liver.

Absorption is the process by which tiny nutrient particles of digested food pass through the intestinal walls into the blood and lymph vessels, which help distribute them to the cells of the body.

The bowels *eliminate* as feces whatever food substances they cannot digest or absorb, such as the plant fiber *cellulose*. Fecal matter also contains bile, which carries the waste products resulting from the breakdown (catabolism) of red blood cells. Nearly one-third of the excreted fecal matter is made up of dead intestinal bacteria. The body can function smoothly and efficiently only if the bowel removes these daily-generated waste products every day.

Good health results when each of these major activities in the digestive system is balanced and well coordinated with the rest of the body. By contrast, abnormalities begin to arise in the digestive system as well as in other parts of the body when one or more of these functions becomes impaired. The presence of gallstones in the liver and gallbladder has a disruptive influence on the digestion and absorption of food, as well as on the body's waste disposal system.

Diseases of the Mouth

Gallstones in the liver and gallbladder are also responsible for most diseases of the mouth. The stones interfere with the digestion and absorption of food, which, in turn, forces waste products meant for elimination to remain in the intestinal tract. The storage of waste in the intestines creates a toxic, anaerobic environment that supports breeding of destructive germs and parasites and undermines preservation of healthy, resilient tissues.

Bacterial infection **(thrush)** and viral infection **(herpes)** in the mouth occur only when the intestines have accumulated considerable amounts of undigested waste matter. Destructive bacteria attempt to decompose some of the waste, but not without producing powerful toxins. Some of these toxins are absorbed into the blood and lymph fluids, which carry them to the liver. The rest of the toxins remain trapped in the intestines where they are a constant source of irritation to the intestinal lining (which begins in the mouth and ends in the anus). Eventually, the intestinal wall becomes inflamed and develops ulcerous lesions. The damaged intestinal tissue begins to "invite" more and more microbes to the scene of injury to help destroy and dispose of any weak and damaged cells. We call this "infection."

Infection is a normal phenomenon seen everywhere in nature whenever there is something that needs to be decomposed. Bacteria never attack—that is, infect something that is as clean, vital, and healthy as a well-nourished fruit hanging on a tree. Only when the fruit becomes overripe, lacks nourishment, or falls to the ground can bacteria begin their clean-up job. While decomposing food or flesh, bacteria produce toxins. You can recognize these toxins by their unpleasant odor and acidic nature. The same occurs when bacteria act on improperly digested food in the intestines. If this situation takes place day after day and month after month, the resulting toxins will lead to symptoms of illness.

Thrush indicates the presence of large quantities of bacteria that have spread throughout the gastrointestinal tract (GI tract), including the mouth area. It shows up in the mouth because the mucus lining there is not as developed and resistant as in the lower parts of the GI tract. The main source of thrush, though, is in the intestines. Since the largest part of the immune system in the body is located in the mucus lining of the GI tract, thrush indicates a major weakness in the body's general immunity to disease.

Herpes, which doctors consider a viral disease, is similar to thrush, with the exception that, instead of bacteria attacking the cell exterior, viral materials attack the nucleus, or cell interior. In both cases, the "attackers" target only weak and unhealthy cells— that is, cells that are already damaged or dysfunctional and are susceptible to mutate into cancerous cells. Added to this survival drama, gallstones can harbor quantities of bacteria and viruses, which escape the liver via the secreted bile and affect those parts of the body that are the least protected or already weakened. The thing to keep in mind is that germs do not infect the body unless it requires their help. The intestinal tract needs bile to keep itself neat and clean. Lack of bile in the intestines prevents this from happening. The next best solution to removing harmful waste matter is to employ destructive germs.

Gallstones can also lead to other problems in the mouth. They inhibit proper bile secretion, which, in turn, reduces appetite and secretions of saliva from the salivary glands in the mouth. Saliva is required to cleanse the mouth and keep its tissues soft and pliable. If not enough saliva is present, destructive bacteria begin to invade the mouth cavity. This can lead to **tooth decay, gum destruction,** and other tooth-related problems. However, to reiterate the previously made point, bacteria do not cause tooth decay. These germs are attracted only to those areas in the mouth that are already congested, undernourished, and acidified.

A **bitter taste** in the mouth is caused by bile that has regurgitated into the stomach and, from there, into the mouth. This condition occurs because of major intestinal congestion, as seen, for example, during bouts of constipation. Instead of properly moving downward and out of the body, parts of the intestinal content back up, which, in turn, may force bile, bacteria, gas, toxins, and other irritating substances into the upper regions of the GI tract. Bile in the mouth, for example, drastically alters the pH-value (acid-alkaline balance) of saliva, which inhibits its cleansing action and makes the mouth susceptible to infectious germs.

A **mouth ulcer** in the lower lip indicates a similar inflammatory process in the large intestine. A repeated occurrence of ulcers (in either one of the two corners of the mouth) points to the presence of **duodenal ulcers** (also see the following section, *Diseases of the Stomach*). **Tongue ulcers,** depending on their location, indicate pockets of inflammation in corresponding areas of the alimentary canal, such as the stomach, small intestine, appendix, or large intestine.

Diseases of the Stomach

As already indicated, gallstones and subsequent digestive trouble can lead to regurgitation of bile and bile salts into the stomach. Such an occurrence adversely changes the composition of gastric juices and the amount of mucus generated in the stomach. The mucus is there to protect the surface stomach lining from the destructive effects of hydrochloric acid. The condition where this protective "shield" is broken or diminished is known as **gastritis.**

Gastritis can occur in acute or chronic form. When the surface cells (epithelium) of the stomach are exposed to acidic gastric juice, the cells absorb hydrogen ions. This increases their internal acidity, counterbalances their basic metabolic processes, and causes an inflammatory reaction. In more severe cases, there may be ulceration of the *mucosa* **(peptic or gastric ulcer),** bleeding, perforation of the stomach wall, and **peritonitis,** a condition that occurs when an ulcer erodes through the full thickness of the stomach or duodenum and their contents enter the peritoneal cavity.

Duodenal ulcers develop when acid leaving the stomach erodes the duodenum's lining. In many cases, the acid production is unusually high. Eating too many foods that require strong acid secretions, as well as improper food combining (for more details see *Timeless Secrets of Health and Rejuvenation* by the author), often disturb balanced acid production. **Esophageal reflux,** commonly known as "heartburn," is a condition in which stomach acid washes upward into the esophagus and causes irritation or injury to the delicate tissues lining the esophagus. Contrary to common opinion, this condition is not due to the stomach's making too much hydrochloric acid, but due instead to back-flushing of waste, toxins, and bile from the intestines into the stomach. In many cases, heartburn results when the stomach makes too little hydrochloric acid, thereby forcing food to remain there far too long and to ferment. Taking antacids can further impair the digestion of foods and cause major damage to the stomach and the rest of the GI tract.

A number of other causes of gastritis and heartburn can be identified. They include overeating, consuming fried foods, excessive alcohol consumption, heavy cigarette smoking, drinking coffee every day, ingesting soda, eating large quantities of animal protein and animal fats, and subjecting oneself to x-radiation, cytotoxic drugs, aspirin, and other anti-inflammatory drugs. Food poisoning, highly spicy foods, iced beverages, dehydration, and emotional stress also cause gastric distress. All of these also cause gallstones in the liver and gallbladder, thereby starting off a vicious cycle and creating major disruptions throughout the GI tract. In the final event, malignant **stomach tumors** may be formed.

Most medical doctors now believe that a "bug" (H. pylori) causes stomach ulcers. Combating the bug with antibiotic drugs usually brings relief and stops the ulcer. Although the drug does not prevent the ulcer from returning after discontinuation, there is a high "recovery" rate. Still, such "recoveries" may cause side effects that are often serious.

The infection by the H. pylori bug is only possible because factors other than a normally harmless germ have already weakened and damaged the stomach cells. In a healthy stomach, the same bug turns out to be completely innocuous. Most of us have lived with this bug without ever being troubled by it. This brings up an important question: Why does the same bug cause an ulcer in some people and not in others? As mentioned before, gallstones in the liver and gallbladder can cause intestinal congestion and thereby lead to frequent back-flushing of bile and toxins into the stomach, which may injure an ever-increasing number of stomach cells. Antibiotics destroy the natural stomach flora, including those bacteria that normally help to break down damaged cells. Although the antibiotic approach results in a quick relief of symptoms, it also lowers stomach performance permanently, which sets up the body for more severe challenges than just dealing with an ulcer.[4] Shortcuts to healing rarely pay off. On the other hand, most stomach disorders disappear spontaneously when all existing gallstones are removed and a healthy diet and balanced lifestyle are followed regularly.

Diseases of the Pancreas

The pancreas is a small gland with its head lying in the curve of the duodenum. Its main duct joins the common bile duct to form what is known as the *ampulla* of the bile duct. The ampulla enters

---

[4] For more details on the treatments of stomach ulcers and their consequences, see the author's book *Timeless Secrets of Health and Rejuvenation.*

the duodenum at its midpoint. Apart from secreting the hormones *insulin* and *glucagon,* the pancreas produces *pancreatic juice,* which contains enzymes that digest carbohydrates, proteins, and fats. When the acidic contents from the stomach enter the duodenum, they combine with alkaline pancreatic juice and bile. This creates the proper acid-alkaline balance (pH-value) at which the pancreatic enzymes are most effective.

Gallstones in the liver or gallbladder cut bile secretions from the normal amount of one quart or more per day, to as little as one cup or less per day. This severely disrupts the digestive process, particularly when fats or fat-containing foods are consumed. Subsequently, the duodenal pH remains too low, which inhibits the action of pancreatic enzymes, as well as those secreted by the small intestine. The net result is that food is only partially digested. Improperly digested food that is saturated with the stomach's hydrochloric acid can have a very irritating, caustic effect on the entire intestinal tract.

If a gallstone has moved from the gallbladder into the ampulla, where the common bile duct and the pancreatic ducts combine (see **Figure 3**), the release of pancreatic juice becomes obstructed and bile moves into the pancreas. This causes a number of protein-splitting pancreatic enzymes, which are normally activated only in the duodenum, to be activated while still in the pancreas. This makes these enzymes highly destructive. They begin to digest parts of the pancreatic tissue, which can lead to infection, suppuration, and local thrombosis. This condition is known as **pancreatitis.**

Gallstones obstructing the ampulla release bacteria, viruses, and toxins into the pancreas, which can cause further damage to pancreatic cells, and eventually lead to **malignant tumors.** The tumors occur mostly in the head of the pancreas, where they inhibit the flow of bile and pancreatic juice. This condition is often accompanied by **jaundice** (for more details see *Diseases of the Liver* below).

Gallstones in the liver, gallbladder, and ampulla may also be partly responsible for both types of **diabetes:** insulin-dependent and non-insulin-dependent. All patients of mine with diagnosed diabetes, including children, have had large quantities of stones in their liver. Each liver flush further improved their condition, provided that they followed a healthy daily regimen and diet void of animal products.[5]

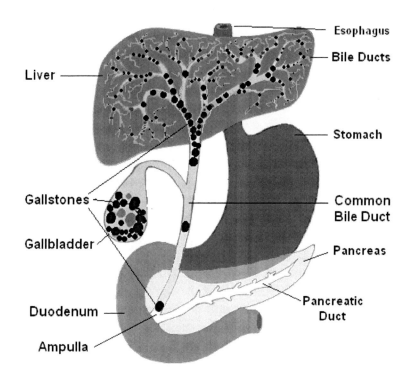

Esophagus

Bile Ducts

Liver

Stomach

Gallstones

Common
Bile Duct

Gallbladder

Pancreas

Duodenum

Pancreatic
Duct

Ampulla

Figure 3: Gallstones in the liver and gallbladder

Diseases of the Liver

The liver is the largest gland/organ in the body. It weighs up to three pounds, is suspended behind the ribs on the upper right side of the abdomen, and spans almost the entire width of the body. Being responsible for hundreds of different functions, it is also the most complex and active organ in the body.

Since the liver is in charge of processing, converting, distributing, and maintaining the body's vital "fuel" supply (for

---

[5] Also see "Overeating Protein" in Chapter 3, and the chapter on diabetes in the author's book *Timeless Secrets of Health and Rejuvenation,* or in *Diabetes—No More!* .

example, nutrients and energy), anything that interferes with these functions must have a serious, detrimental impact on the health of the liver and the body as a whole. The strongest interference stems from the presence of gallstones.

Besides manufacturing cholesterol—an essential building material of organ cells, hormones, and bile—the liver also produces hormones and proteins that affect the way the body functions, grows, and heals. Furthermore, it makes new amino acids[6] and converts existing ones into proteins. These proteins are the main building blocks of the cells, hormones, neurotransmitters, genes, and so forth. Other essential functions of the liver include breaking down old, worn-out cells; recycling proteins and iron; and storing vitamins and nutrients. Gallstones are a hazard to all these vital tasks.

In addition to breaking down alcohol in the blood, the liver also detoxifies noxious substances, bacteria, parasites, and certain components of pharmaceutical drugs. It uses specific enzymes to convert waste or poisons into substances that can be safely removed from the body. In addition, the liver filters more than one quart of blood each minute. Most of the filtered waste products leave the liver via the bile stream. Gallstones obstructing the bile ducts lead to high levels of toxicity in the liver and, ultimately, to **liver diseases.** This development is further exacerbated by one's intake of pharmaceutical drugs, normally broken down by the liver. The presence of gallstones prevents their detoxification, which can cause "overdosing" and devastating side effects, even at normal doses. It also means that the liver is at risk for damage from the breakdown products of the drugs on which it acts. Alcohol that is not detoxified properly by the liver can seriously injure or destroy liver cells.

All liver diseases are preceded by extensive bile duct obstruction through gallstones. The gallstones distort the structural framework of the *liver lobules* (see **Figures 3 and 4**), which are the main units constituting the liver (which contains more than 50,000 such units). Subsequently, blood circulation to and from these lobules, and the cells of which they are composed, becomes

---

[6] Right from a baby's first breath, the body produces amino acids and proteins from the nitrogen, carbon, oxygen, and hydrogen molecules contained in the air.

increasingly difficult. In addition, the liver cells have to cut down bile production. Nerve fibers also become damaged. Prolonged suffocation due to the presence of stones eventually damages or destroys liver cells and their lobules. Fibrous tissue gradually replaces damaged cells, causing further obstruction and an increase in pressure on the liver's blood vessels. If the regeneration of liver cells does not keep pace with this damage, **liver cirrhosis** is imminent. Liver cirrhosis usually leads to death.

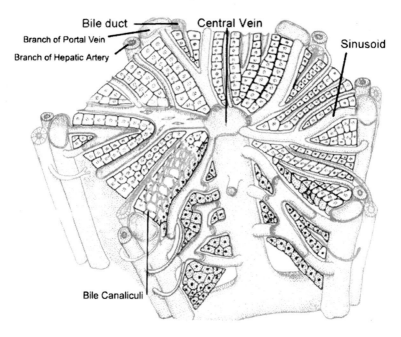

Figure 4: A liver lobule

Liver failure occurs when cell suffocation destroys so many liver cells that the number of cells required to carry out the organ's most important and vital functions is insufficient. Consequences of liver failure include drowsiness, confusion, shaking of hands tremor, drop in blood sugar, infection, kidney failure and fluid retention, uncontrolled bleeding, coma, and death. The capability of the liver to recover from major damage, though, is truly remarkable. Once the liver flush has removed all gallstones, and the afflicted person discontinues using alcohol and medicinal drugs, there usually are no significant long-term consequences, even though many of the liver cells may have been destroyed during the illness. When the cells grow again, they will do so in an ordered fashion that permits normal liver functions. This is possible because in liver failure (as opposed to liver cirrhosis) the basic structure of the liver has not been substantially compromised.

Acute **hepatitis** results when whole groups of liver cells begin to die off. Gallstones harbor large quantities of viral material, which can invade and infect liver cells, causing cell-degenerative changes. As gallstones increase in number and size, and as more cells become infected and die, entire lobules begin to collapse, and blood vessels begin to develop kinks. This greatly affects blood circulation to the remaining liver cells. The extent of the damage that these changes have on the liver and its overall performance largely depends on the degree of obstruction caused by the gallstones in the liver bile ducts. Cancer of the liver only occurs after many years of progressive occlusion of the liver bile ducts. This applies also to tumors in the liver that emanate from primary tumors in the GI tract, lungs, or breast.

Most **liver infections** (type A, type B, type non-A, and type non-B) occur when a certain number of liver lobules are congested with gallstones, which can even happen at a very early age. The now common practice of prematurely cutting or clamping the umbilical cord that connects a newborn baby with his mother, leaves the child with just two-thirds of its required blood volume, a lot of toxins normally filtered out by the placenta during the first hour after birth, and nearly no antibodies to protect it against disease. It usually takes at least 40 to 60 minutes before the umbilical cord stops throbbing completely. Cutting the cord too early constitutes an act of medical negligence that can affect the baby's liver right from the start and set it up for gallstone formation even during childhood. This can subsequently lead to liver infections.

A healthy liver and immune system are perfectly able to destroy viral material, regardless of whether the virus has been picked up from the external environment or has entered the bloodstream in some other way. The majority of all people exposed to these viruses never fall ill. In fact, we all have most viruses that exist outside the body in our body right now. However, when large amounts of gallstones are present, the liver becomes congested and toxic, which turns it into a conducive environment for viral activity. Viruses are intracellular parasites that enter a host cell and take over the host's cellular machinery to produce new viral particles (it also has been proved that viruses can be created from bacteria within the cells). But viruses don't develop and attack cells randomly. Contrary to common belief, viruses tend to "hijack" the nuclei of the weakest and most damaged cells to prevent them from mutating. Not all viruses succeed, though, and liver cancer may result. Their presence in cancer cells should not be misconstrued to have cancer-producing effects.

Gallstones can harbor plenty of live viruses. Some of these viruses break free and enter the blood. This is known as chronic hepatitis. Nonviral infections of the liver may be triggered (not caused) by bacteria that spread from any of the bile ducts obstructed with gallstones.

The presence of gallstones in the bile ducts also impairs the liver cells' ability to deal with toxic substances such as chloroform, cytotoxic drugs, anabolic steroids, alcohol, aspirin, fungi, food additives, and the like. When this occurs, the body develops hypersensitivity to these predictable toxic substances and to other unpredictable ones contained in numerous medicinal drugs. Many **allergies** stem from such conditions of hypersensitivity. For the same reason, there may also be a drastic increase in toxic side effects resulting from the intake of medicinal drugs, side effects that the Food and Drug Administration (FDA) or pharmaceutical companies may not even be aware of.

The most common form of **jaundice** results from gallstones being stuck in the bile duct leading to the duodenum, and/or from gallstones and fibrous tissue distorting the structural framework of the liver lobules. The movement of bile through the bile channels (canaliculi) is blocked, and the liver cells can no longer conjugate[7] and excrete bile pigment, known as *bilirubin*. Consequently, there is a buildup in the bloodstream of both bile and the substances from which it is made. As bilirubin begins to build up in the blood,

---

[7] Conjugation is a biochemical process to bind a substance to an acid, and thereby deactivating its biological activity, making it water-soluble, and facilitating its excretion.

it stains the skin. Bilirubin concentration in the blood may be three times above normal before a **yellow coloration** of both the skin and the conjunctiva of the eyes becomes apparent. Unconjugated bilirubin has a toxic effect on brain cells. A tumor in the head of the pancreas caused by bile duct congestion may also cause jaundice.

Diseases of the Gallbladder and Bile Ducts

The liver secretes bile, which passes via the two hepatic ducts into the common hepatic duct. The common hepatic duct runs for 1.5 inches before joining the cystic duct that connects it with the gallbladder. Liver bile continues its journey through the common bile duct into the intestinal tract, but most of it must first pass into the gallbladder. The gallbladder is a pear-shaped pouch that protrudes from the bile duct. It is attached to the posterior side of the liver (see **Figure 5**).

A normal gallbladder generally holds about 2 fluid ounces of bile. The bile stored in the gallbladder, however, has a different consistency than the bile found in the liver. In the gallbladder, most of the salt and water contained in the bile is reabsorbed, thus reducing its volume to a mere one- tenth of its original quantity. Bile salts (as opposed to regular salt) are not absorbed, though, which means their concentration is increased about tenfold. On the other hand, the gallbladder adds mucus to the bile, which turns it into a thick, mucus-like substance. Its high concentration makes bile the powerful digestive aid that it is.

The muscular walls of the gallbladder contract and eject bile when acidic foods and most protein foods enter the duodenum from the stomach. A more marked gallbladder activity is noted if food entering the duodenum contains a high proportion of fat. The body uses the bile salts contained in bile to emulsify the fat and facilitate its digestion. Once the bile salts have done their job and left the emulsified fat for intestinal absorption, they travel on down the intestine. Most of them are reabsorbed in the final section of the small intestine (ileum) and carried back to the liver. Once in the liver, the bile salts are collected again in the bile and secreted into the duodenum. Intestinal congestion sharply reduces the amount of bile salts needed for proper bile production and fat digestion. Diminished bile salt concentration in the bile causes gallstones, and leaves large amounts of fats undigested; this is hazardous to the intestinal environment.

Gallstones in the gallbladder may be made primarily of cholesterol, calcium, or pigments such as bilirubin. Cholesterol is the commonest component, but many of the stones are of mixed composition. Besides the above ingredients, gallstones may contain bile salts, water, and mucus, as well as toxins, bacteria, and, sometimes, dead parasites.

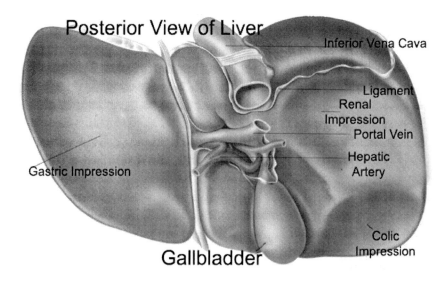

Figure 5: Location of the gallbladder

Typically, stones in the gallbladder keep growing in size for about eight years before noticeable symptoms begin to appear. Larger stones are generally calcified and can be detected easily through radiological means or by using *ultrasound*. Some 85 percent of the gallstones found in the gallbladder measure about ¾ inches across (see **Figure 6a**), although some can become as large as 2 to 3 inches across (see **Figure 6b** of a calcified gallstone; I personally examined and photographed this stone moments after my wife released it without any pain during her ninth liver flush; the stone emitted an extremely noxious odor unlike any I had ever come across). Such stones form when, for reasons explained in Chapter

3, bile in the gallbladder becomes too saturated and its unabsorbed constituents begin to harden.

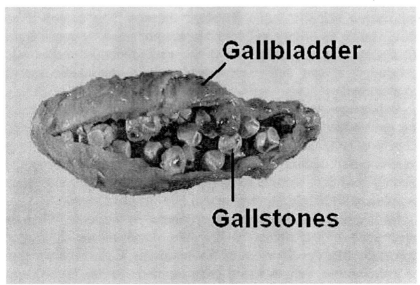

Figure 6a: Gallstones in a dissected gallbladder

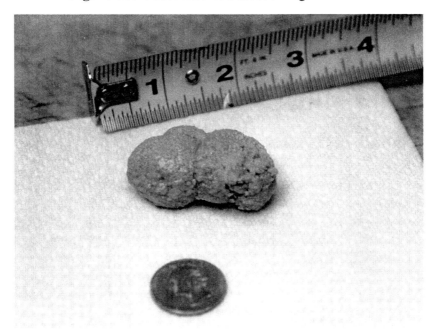

Figure 6b: A large calcified gallstone, passed painlessly

If a gallstone slips out of the gallbladder and becomes impacted in the *cystic bile duct* or *common bile duct*, there is very strong spasmodic contraction of the wall of the duct (see **Figure 3**). The contraction helps to move the stone onward. This causes severe pain, known as **biliary colic,** and is accompanied by considerable distension of the gallbladder. If the gallbladder is packed with gallstones, it can suffer extremely painful spasmodic muscle contractions.

Gallstones can cause irritation and inflammation of the lining of the gallbladder, as well as of the cystic and common bile ducts. This is a condition known as **cholecystitis.** There may also be superimposed microbial infection. It is quite common to encounter ulceration of the tissues between the gallbladder and the duodenum or colon, with **fistula formation** and **fibrous adhesions.**

Gallbladder disease generally originates in the liver. When the occurrence of gallstones in the bile ducts of the liver and, eventually, the development of fibrous tissue, distort the structure of liver lobules, venous blood pressure starts to rise in the portal vein. This, in turn, increases the blood pressure in the cystic vein, which drains venous blood from the gallbladder into the portal vein. The incomplete elimination of waste products through the cystic duct causes a backup of acidic waste in the tissues composing the gallbladder. This gradually reduces the stamina and performance of the gallbladder. Subsequently, the formation of mineralized gallstones is just a matter of time.

Intestinal Diseases

The small intestine is continuous with the stomach at the *pyloric sphincter* and has a length of 16–19 feet. It leads into the large intestine, which is about 3.5–5 feet long. The small intestine secretes intestinal juice to complete the digestion of carbohydrates, proteins, and fats. It also absorbs nutrient materials necessary for nourishing and maintaining the body and protects it against infection by microbes that have survived the antimicrobial action of hydrochloric acid in the stomach.

When acid food (*chyme*) from the stomach enters the duodenum, it combines first with bile and pancreatic juice, and then with intestinal juice. Gallstones in the liver and gallbladder drastically reduce the secretion of bile, which weakens the ability of *pancreatic enzymes* to digest carbohydrates, proteins, and fats. This, in turn, prevents the small intestine from properly absorbing the nutrient components of these foods (such as *monosaccharides* from carbohydrates, *amino acids* from protein, and *fatty acids* and *glycerol* from fats). This incomplete absorption can lead to malnourishment and food cravings.

Since the presence of bile in the intestines is essential for the absorption of life-essential fats, calcium, and vitamin K, gallstones can lead to life-threatening diseases, such as **heart disease, osteoporosis,** and **cancer.** The liver uses the fat-soluble vitamin K to produce the compounds responsible for the clotting of blood. In case of poor vitamin K absorption, **hemorrhagic disease** may result. The body cannot fully absorb this vitamin when a problem with the digestion of fat exists. The main cause of inadequate vitamin K absorption is an insufficient supply of bile, pancreatic lipase, and pancreatic fat. It stands to reason that following a low-fat or no-fat diet can actually endanger your life.

Calcium is essential for the hardening of bone and teeth, the coagulation of blood, and the mechanism of muscle contraction. Poor bile secretion can, therefore, undermine the uptake of calcium, a mineral the body requires for some of its most vital activities.

What applies to vitamin K also applies to all other fat-soluble vitamins, including vitamins A, E, and D. The small intestine can only absorb vitamin A and carotene sufficiently if fat absorption is normal. If vitamin A absorption is insufficient, the *epithelial cells* become damaged. These cells form an essential part of all the organs, blood vessels, lymph vessels, and so on in the body. Vitamin A is also necessary to maintain healthy eyes and protect against or reduce microbial infection. Vitamin D is essential for calcification of bones and teeth.[8] It is of great importance to realize

---

[8] The only truly safe way to get enough vitamin D is from exposure to sunlight and certain foods. See more details in the chapter "Sunlight—Medicine of Nature" of the author's book *Timeless Secrets of Health and Rejuvenation*.

that supplementing these vitamins does not resolve the problem of deficiency.[9]

To sum up, without normal bile secretions, the body cannot digest and absorb enough of these vitamins, which, in turn, can cause considerable damage to the circulatory, lymphatic, and urinary systems.

Inadequately digested foods tend to ferment and putrefy in the small and large intestines. They attract a vast number of bacteria to help speed up the process of decomposition. The breakdown products are often very toxic, and so are the excretions produced by the bacteria. All of this strongly irritates the mucus lining, which is one of the body's foremost defense lines against disease-causing agents. Regular exposure to these toxins impairs the body's immune system, 60 percent of which is located in the intestines. Overburdened by a constant invasion of toxins, the small and large intestines may be afflicted with a number of disorders, including **diarrhea, constipation, abdominal gas, Crohn's disease, ulcerative colitis, diverticular disease, hernias, polyps, dysentery, appendicitis, volvulus,** and **intussusceptions,** as well as both **benign** and **malignant tumors.**

Ample bile flow maintains good digestion and absorption of food and has a strong cleansing action throughout the intestinal tract. Every part of the body depends on the basic nutrients made available through the digestive system, as well as the efficient removal of waste products from that system. Gallstones in the liver and gallbladder considerably disrupt both these vital processes. Therefore, they can be held accountable for most, if not all, of the different kinds of ailments that can afflict the body. Removal of gallstones helps to normalize the digestive and eliminative functions, improve cell metabolism, and maintain balance throughout the body.

---

[9] See details on the vitamin issue in *Timeless Secrets of Health and Rejuvenation.*

Disorders of the Circulatory System

For descriptive reasons, I have divided the *circulatory system* into two main parts, the *blood circulatory system* and the *lymphatic system*. The blood circulatory system consists of the heart, which acts as a pump, and the blood vessels, through which the blood circulates.

The lymphatic system consists of lymph nodes and lymph vessels, through which colorless *lymph* flows. The body contains three times more lymph fluid than blood. Lymph takes up waste products from the cells, as well as cellular debris, and removes these from the body.

The lymphatic system is the primary circulatory system used by all immunological cells: macrophages, T-cells, B-cells, lymphocytes, and so forth. An obstruction-free lymphatic system is necessary to maintain strong immunity and homeostasis.

Coronary Heart Disease

Heart attacks take more American lives than any other cause. Although it occurs suddenly, a heart attack is actually the final stage of an insidious disorder that has been years in the making. This disorder is known as coronary heart disease. Since the disease plunders mostly prosperous nations and rarely killed anyone before 1900, we have to hold our modern lifestyle, unnatural foods, and unbalanced eating habits responsible for today's literally heartsick society. However, long before the heart begins to malfunction, the liver loses much of its major vitality and efficiency.

The liver influences the entire circulatory system, including the heart. In fact, the liver is the greatest protector of the heart. Under normal conditions, the liver thoroughly detoxifies and purifies venous blood that arrives via the portal vein from the abdominal part of the digestive system, the spleen, and the pancreas. In addition to breaking down alcohol, the liver detoxifies noxious substances, such as toxins produced by microbes. It also kills bacteria and parasites and neutralizes certain drug compounds with the help of specific enzymes. One of the liver's most ingenious feats is to remove the nitrogenous portion of amino acids, since nitrogen is not required for the formation of new protein. It forms *urea* from this waste product. The urea ends up in the bloodstream and is excreted in the urine. The liver also breaks down the nucleoprotein (nucleus) of worn-out cells of the body. The byproduct of this process is *uric acid*, which is excreted with the urine as well.

The liver filters more than one quart of blood per minute, leaving only the acidic carbon dioxide for elimination through the lungs (see **Figure 7**).

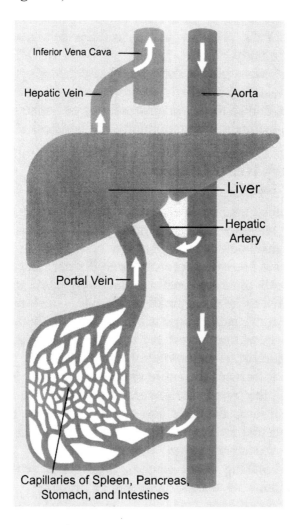

Figure 7: The way the liver filters blood

After it is purified in the liver, the blood passes through the *hepatic vein* into the *inferior vena cava,* which takes it straight into the right side of the heart. From there the venous blood is carried to the lungs, where the interchange of gases takes place: carbon dioxide is excreted and oxygen absorbed. After leaving the lungs, the oxygenated blood passes into the left side of the heart. From there it is pumped into the *aorta,* which supplies all body tissues with oxygenated blood.

Gallstones in the bile ducts of the liver distort the basic framework of the lobules. Consequently, the blood vessels supplying these liver units develop kinks, which greatly reduces internal blood supply. Liver cells become damaged, and harmful cellular debris begins to enter the bloodstream. This further weakens the liver's ability to detoxify the blood. As a result, more and more harmful substances are retained both in the liver and in the blood. A congested liver can obstruct the venous blood flow to the heart, leading to heart palpitations or even heart attacks. It is obvious that toxins that are not neutralized by the liver end up damaging the heart and blood vessel network.

Another consequence of this development is that proteins from dead cells (about 30 billion cells per day) and unused food proteins are not sufficiently broken down, which, in turn, raises protein concentrations in the blood. As a result, the body tries to store these proteins in the basal membranes of the blood vessel walls (further explanation of this scenario is provided below). Once the body's storage capacity for protein is exhausted, any new proteins taken up by the blood remain trapped in the bloodstream. This can cause the number of red blood cells to increase, which raises the packed cell volume of the blood, called *hemocrit,* to abnormal levels. ·At the same time, the concentration of *hemoglobin* in the blood begins to increase, which may give rise to a red complexion of the skin, particularly in the face and chest. (*Note:* Hemoglobin is a complex protein that combines with oxygen in the lungs and transports it to all body cells.) As a result, the red blood cells become enlarged and are, therefore, too big to pass through the tiny vessels of the capillary network. Evidently, this causes the blood to become too thick and slow moving, thereby increasing its tendency toward clotting (platelets sticking together).

The formation of blood clots is considered to be the main risk factor for **heart attack** or **stroke.** Since fat has no clotting ability, this risk stems mainly from the high concentration of protein in the blood. Researchers have discovered that the sulphur-containing amino acid *homocysteine* (HC) promotes the tiny clots that initiate arterial damage and the catastrophic ones that precipitate most heart attacks and strokes (Ann Clin & Lab Sci 1991; Lancet 1981). Be aware that HC is up to forty times more predictive than cholesterol in assessing cardiovascular disease risk. HC results from the normal metabolism of the amino acid *methionine*—which is abundant in red meat, milk, and dairy products. High concentrations of protein in the blood hinder the continuously required distribution of important nutrients, especially water, glucose, and oxygen to the cells. Excessive amounts of proteins in the blood are also responsible for blood dehydration, that is, blood thickening—one of the leading causes of high blood pressure and heart disease. Furthermore, these proteins undermine complete elimination of basic metabolic waste products (see section below on *Poor Circulation...*). All these factors combined coerce the body to raise its blood pressure. This condition, which is commonly known as **hypertension,** reduces the life-endangering effect of blood thickening, to some extent. It also permits enough nutrient-rich blood to circulate through the congested body. However, this life-saving response to a life-threatening situation unduly stresses and damages the blood vessels. This may still be a better scenario, though, than the one that occurs when the blood pressure is lowered through medication. Leading health experts now recognize hypertensive drugs to be a major cause of congestive heart failure and other debilitating illnesses. Congestive heart failure is a progressive condition of "dying very slowly" whereby every small movement, every breath taken, and every word uttered take huge efforts, and the body becomes unable to perform even the simplest of tasks.

One of the body's first and most efficient approaches for avoiding the danger of an imminent heart attack is to take excessive proteins out of the bloodstream and store them elsewhere, for the time being (see **Figure 8**).

Thickening of Blood Capillary Wall

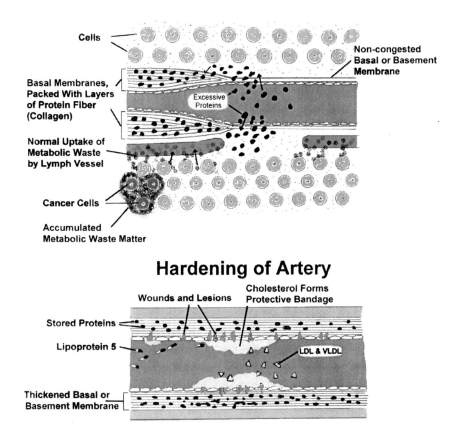

Figure 8: The beginning stages of heart disease

The only place where protein can be accommodated in large quantities is the blood vessel network. The capillary walls are able to absorb most of the excessive, unused, or unusable protein. The body converts the soluble protein into *collagen fiber,* which is 100 percent protein, and stores it in the *basal membrane* of the blood vessel walls. The basal membrane has the capacity to increase its thickness by eight to ten times before its storage capacity for protein is exhausted. Storing proteins in the blood vessel walls also means that the body can no longer pass adequate amounts of oxygen, glucose, and other essential nutrients to the cells. The cells affected by such a "famine" may include those that make up the heart muscle. The result is **heart muscle weakness** and reduced performance of the heart. This, in turn, contributes to degenerative illnesses, including diabetes, fibromyalgia, arthritis, and cancer. Whenever the heart is affected, the entire body suffers.

Once the capillary walls have no space left to accommodate excessive protein, the basal membranes of the arteries themselves start taking up protein. The beneficial effect of this action is that the blood remains thin enough to avert the threat of a heart attack, at least for some time. Eventually, though, the very same tactic that prevents the threat of sudden death also damages the blood vessel walls. (*Note:* Only the more primary survival mechanisms of the body, such as the fight-or-flight response, the common cold, or diarrhea, are without significant side effects.) The inner lining of the arterial walls becomes rough and thick, like rust in a water pipe. Cracks, wounds, and lesions appear at various locations.

Smaller blood vessel injuries are dealt with by *blood platelets.* These tiny blood components release the hormone *serotonin,* which helps to constrict the blood vessels and reduce bleeding. However, larger wounds, as are typically found in diseased coronary arteries, cannot be sealed by platelets alone; they require the body's more complex process of blood clotting. If a blood clot breaks loose, it can enter the heart and result in **myocardial infarction,** commonly called a heart attack. A clot that reaches the brain results in a stroke. A blood clot entering the opening of a pulmonary artery that delivers used blood to the lungs can be fatal.

To prevent this danger before it arises, the body uses an entire arsenal of first aid measures, including the release of the blood chemical *lipoprotein 5* (LP5) and cholesterol. Owing to it sticky nature, LP5 works as a "Band-Aid" to create a firmer seal around the wounds and lesions within the arteries.

As a secondary but equally important rescue operation, the body attaches specific types of cholesterol to the injured areas of an artery (more on this in the section "High Cholesterol"). This acts as a more reliable bandage than LP5 can provide. Since cholesterol deposits still are not protection or fortification enough, extra connective tissue and smooth muscle cells begin to grow inside the blood vessel.

Called atherosclerotic plaques, these deposits can eventually block an artery completely, thereby severely obstructing the flow of blood to the heart. In response to this grave situation—unless interfered with through a bypass operation, angioplasty, or the insertion of a stent—the body makes its own bypasses by turning existing or new capillaries into small, blood-supplying arteries. Although this option is better than surgery, it still does not significantly reduce the danger of a heart attack.

Contrary to common assumption, a heart attack does not occur as a result of blood vessel obstruction, but rather because of blood clots and/or soft fragments of atherosclerotic deposits making their way into the heart. The blood clots and soft pieces of cholesterol implicated in triggering heart attacks are almost never released from the rock-hard structures of the more occluded sections of an artery, but tend to be released from newly created lesions and their protective cholesterol patches. For this reason, stent or bypass operations have neither reduced the incidence of heart attacks nor lowered the mortality rate from these attacks.

Although the gradual destruction of blood vessels, known as **atherosclerosis,** initially protects a person's life against a heart attack caused by a blood clot, it is eventually also responsible for causing such an attack. Most forms of coronary heart disease can be reversed by cleansing the liver and by clearing out any existing protein deposits in the capillaries and arteries. (See Chapter 3.)

High Cholesterol

Cholesterol is an important building block of every cell in the body and is essential for all metabolic processes. It is particularly important in the production of nerve tissue, bile, and hormones. On the average, our body produces about half a gram to one gram of cholesterol per day, depending on how much of it the body needs at the time. The adult human body is able to produce 400 times more cholesterol per day than what it would obtain from eating 3.5 ounces of butter. The main cholesterol producers are the liver and the small intestine, in that order. Normally, they are able to release cholesterol directly into the bloodstream, where it is instantly tied to blood proteins. These proteins, which are called lipoproteins, are in charge of transporting the cholesterol to its numerous destinations. Three main types of lipoproteins are in charge of transporting cholesterol: *low density lipoprotein* (LDL), *very low density lipoprotein* (VLDL), and *high density lipoprotein* (HDL).

In comparison to HDL, which researchers privileged with the name "good" cholesterol, LDL and VLDL are both relatively large cholesterol molecules; in fact, they are the richest in cholesterol. There is good reason for their large size. Unlike their smaller cousin, which easily passes through blood vessel walls, the LDL and VLDL versions of cholesterol are meant to take a different pathway; they leave the bloodstream in the liver.

The blood vessels supplying the liver have a quite different structure than the ones supplying other parts of the body. They are known as *sinusoids*. Their unique, grid-like structure permits the liver cells to receive the entire blood content, including the larger cholesterol molecules. The liver cells rebuild the cholesterol and excrete it, along with bile, into the intestines. Once the cholesterol enters the intestines, it combines with fats, is absorbed by the lymph, and enters the blood, in that order. Gallstones in the bile ducts of the liver inhibit bile secretion and partially, or even completely, block the cholesterol's escape route. Owing to backup pressure on the liver cells, bile production drops. Typically, a healthy liver produces over a quart of bile per day. When the major bile ducts are blocked, barely a cup of bile, or even less, will find its way to the intestines. This prevents much of the VLDL and LDL cholesterol from being excreted with the bile.

Gallstones in the liver bile ducts distort the structural framework of the liver lobules, which damages and congests the sinusoids. Deposits of excessive protein also close the grid holes of these blood vessels (see more detailed explanations in the previous section or in the book *Timeless Secrets of Health and Rejuvenation*). Whereas the "good" cholesterol HDL has small enough molecules to leave the bloodstream through ordinary capillaries, the larger LDL and VLDL molecules are more or less trapped in the blood. The result is that LDL and VLDL concentrations begin to rise in the blood to levels that seem potentially harmful to the body. Yet even this scenario is merely part of the body's survival tactics. The body needs the extra cholesterol to patch up the increasing number of cracks and wounds that are formed because of the accumulation of excessive protein in the blood vessel walls. Eventually, though, even the life-saving "bad" cholesterol, which rushes to every wound or injured site in the body, cannot completely prevent blood clot formation in a coronary artery, in which event one of the escaping blood clots may enter the heart and cut off its oxygen supply.

In addition to this complication, reduced bile secretion impairs the digestion of food, particularly fats. Therefore, not enough cholesterol is available for basic cell metabolism. Since the liver cells no longer receive sufficient amounts of LDL and VLDL molecules, those liver cells assume that the blood is deficient in these types of cholesterol. This stimulates the liver cells to increase the production of cholesterol, further raising the levels of LDL and VLDL cholesterol in the blood. Hence, the "bad" cholesterol is trapped in the circulatory system because its escape routes, the bile ducts and the liver sinusoids, are blocked or damaged. The arteries attach as much of the "bad" cholesterol to their walls as they possibly can. Consequently, the arterial walls become rigid and hard, which is still better, though, than having all their wounds and lesions exposed to the gushing blood stream.

Coronary heart disease, regardless of whether it is caused by smoking, drinking excessive amounts of alcohol, overeating protein foods, stress, or any other factor, usually does not occur unless gallstones have impacted the bile ducts of the liver. Removing gallstones from the liver and gallbladder cannot only prevent a heart attack or stroke, but can also help reverse coronary heart disease and heart muscle damage. Cholesterol levels begin to normalize as the distorted and damaged liver lobules regenerate themselves.

Cholesterol-lowering drugs (statins) don't bring the body back to a healthful condition in which the liver can normalize blood cholesterol. Instead, statins artificially lower the level of cholesterol in the blood by blocking the enzyme in the liver that is responsible for making cholesterol. However, by creating an artificial "cholesterol famine" in the liver, bile is not formed properly, which increases the risk of gallstones and hinders the proper digestion of food. The side effects of statins are numerous; they include kidney failure, liver disease, and yes, heart disease (for more information on statins see *Timeless Secrets of Health and Rejuvenation*).

Cholesterol is essential for the normal functioning of the immune system, particularly for the body's response to the millions of cancer cells that every person's body makes each day (the immune system tracks down these cells and kills them through a sophisticated arsenal of weaponry, including the drilling of holes into the cell walls and pumping of a fluid into the cell's interior, causing them to burst and die; for more detailed information about what causes cancer and how to heal it, see Cancer Is Not A Disease – It's A Survival Mechanism).

Despite all the health problems associated with high cholesterol levels, this important substance is *not* something we should try to eliminate from our bodies. Cholesterol does far more good than harm. The harm is generally symptomatic of other problems. I wish to emphasize, once again, that "bad" cholesterol only attaches itself to the walls of arteries to avert immediate heart trouble—not to cause it. The body has no intention to commit suicide, even if doctors like to imply this by the use of suppressive, intervening treatments.

The fact that cholesterol never attaches itself to the walls of veins should be part of the cholesterol discussion. When a doctor tests your cholesterol levels, she takes the blood sample from a vein, not from an artery. Because blood flow is much slower in veins than in arteries, cholesterol should obstruct veins much more readily than arteries, but it never does. There simply is no need for that. Why? Because there are no abrasions and tears in the lining of the vein that require patching up. Cholesterol only affixes itself to arteries in order to coat and cover the abrasions and protect the underlying tissue like a waterproof bandage. Veins do not absorb proteins in their basal membranes like capillaries and arteries do and, therefore, are not prone to this type of injury.

"Bad" cholesterol *saves* lives; it does *not* take lives. LDL allows the blood to flow through injured blood vessels without causing a life-endangering situation. The theory that high LDL is a major cause of coronary heart disease is unproved and unscientific. It has misled the population to believe that cholesterol is an enemy that has to be fought against and destroyed at all costs. Human studies have not shown a cause-and-effect relationship between cholesterol and heart disease. There are hundreds of studies that were intended to prove that such a relationship exists, but all they revealed was a statistical correlation between cholesterol and heart disease—quite fortunately, I might add. If there were no "bad" cholesterol molecules attaching themselves to injured arteries, we would have millions more deaths from heart attack than we already have. By contrast, dozens of conclusive studies have shown that the risk of heart disease increases significantly in people whose HDL levels decrease. It would be much wiser to find out what keeps HDL levels normal than to inhibit cholesterol production in the liver and thereby destroy this precious organ. Elevated LDL cholesterol is not a *cause* of heart disease; rather, it is a *consequence* of an unbalanced liver, of a congested, dehydrated circulatory system, and of a poor diet and lifestyle.

If your doctor has told you that lowering your cholesterol with statins will protect you against heart attacks, you have been grossly misled. The #1 prescribed cholesterol-lowering medicine is Lipitor. I suggest that you read the following warning statement, issued on the official Lipitor web site:

"LIPITOR® (atorvastatin calcium) is a prescription drug used with diet to lower cholesterol. LIPITOR is not for everyone, including those with liver disease or possible liver problems, and women who are nursing, pregnant, or may become pregnant. LIPITOR has not been shown to prevent heart disease or heart attacks."

According to a study published in the *Journal of the American Medical Association*, entitled "Cholesterol and Mortality," after age 50 there is no increased overall death rate associated with high cholesterol. The same study showed that for every 1 mg/dl drop in cholesterol in your body, your risk of death soared by a whopping 14 percent. In other words, taking statins can kill you.

My question is this: Why risk a patient's health or life by giving him a drug that has no effect whatsoever in preventing the problem for which it is being prescribed? The reason why the lowering of cholesterol levels cannot *prevent* heart disease is that cholesterol does not *cause* heart disease. In a recent heart disease study,[10] lowering cholesterol levels was no longer part of the

---

[10] See details of this study in *Timeless Secrets of Health and Rejuvenation.*

recommendations—but try to tell that to statin-prescribing doctors or drug makers!

The most important issue with regard to cholesterol is how efficiently a person's body uses cholesterol and other fats. The body's ability to digest, process, and utilize fats depends on how clear and unobstructed the bile ducts of the liver are. When bile flow is unrestricted and balanced, both the LDL level and the HDL level are balanced as well. Therefore, keeping the bile ducts open is one of the best things you can do to prevent coronary heart disease.

Poor Circulation, Enlargement of the Heart and Spleen, Varicose Veins, Lymph Congestion, Hormonal Imbalances

Gallstones in the liver may lead to poor circulation, enlargement of the heart and spleen, varicose veins, congested lymph vessels, and hormone imbalances. When gallstones have grown large enough to seriously distort the structural framework of the lobules (units) of the liver, blood flow through the liver becomes increasingly difficult. This not only raises the venous blood pressure in the liver, but also raises it in all the organs and areas of the body that drain used blood through their respective veins into the liver's portal vein. Restricted blood flow in that portal vein causes congestion, particularly in the spleen, stomach, esophagus, pancreas, gallbladder, and small and large intestines. This can lead to an enlargement of these organs, to a reduction of their ability to remove cellular waste products, and to a clogging of their respective veins.

A **varicose vein** is one that is so dilated that the valves do not sufficiently close to prevent blood from flowing backward. Sustained pressure on the veins at the junction of the rectum and anus in the large intestine leads to the development of **hemorrhoids,** a type of varicose vein. Other common sites of varicose veins are the legs, the esophagus, and the scrotum.

Dilation of veins and *venules* (small veins) can occur anywhere in the body. It always indicates an obstruction of blood flow.[11]

Poor blood flow through the liver always affects the heart. When the organs of the digestive system become weakened by an increase in venous pressure, they become congested and begin to accumulate harmful waste, including debris from cells that have been broken down. The spleen becomes enlarged while it is dealing with the extra workload associated with removing damaged or worn-out blood cells. This further slows blood circulation to and from the organs of the digestive system, which **stresses the heart, raises blood pressure,** and **injures blood vessels.** The right half of the heart, which receives venous blood via the *inferior vena cava* from the liver and all other parts below the lungs, becomes overloaded with toxic, sometimes infectious, material. This eventually causes enlargement, and possibly infection, of the right side of the heart.

Almost all types of heart disease have one thing in common: blood flow is being obstructed. But blood circulation does not become disrupted easily. It must be preceded by a major congestion of the bile ducts in the liver. Gallstones obstructing the bile ducts dramatically reduce or cut off the blood supply to the liver cells. Reduced blood flow through the liver affects the blood flow in the entire body, which, in turn, has a detrimental effect on the lymphatic system.

The lymphatic system, which is closely linked with the immune system, helps to clear the body of harmful metabolic waste products, foreign material, and cell debris. All cells release metabolic waste products into, and take up nutrients from, a surrounding solution, called *extracellular fluid* or *connective tissue*. The degree of nourishment and efficiency of the cells depends on how swiftly and completely waste material is removed from the extracellular fluid. Since most waste products cannot pass directly into the blood for excretion, they accumulate in the

---

[11] Prescribed by doctors in Germany as a highly successful alternative to surgery for varicose veins, the herbal remedy *horse chestnut seed*, or *conkers,* is very effective in the treatment of "heavy legs," hemorrhoids, and cramps. In combination with cleansing of the liver, colon, and kidneys, conkers can lead to complete recovery.

extracellular fluid until they are removed and detoxified by the lymphatic system. The potentially harmful material is filtered and neutralized by *lymph nodes* that are strategically located throughout the body. One of the key functions of the lymphatic system is to keep the extracellular fluid clear of toxic substances, which makes this a system of utmost importance.

Poor circulation of blood in the body causes an overload of foreign, harmful waste matter in the extracellular tissues and, consequently, in the lymph vessels and lymph nodes as well. When lymph drainage slows down or becomes obstructed, the thymus gland, tonsils, and spleen start to deteriorate quite rapidly. These organs form an important part of the body's system of purification and immunity. In addition, microbes harbored in gallstones can be a constant source of recurring infection in the body, which may render the lymphatic and immune systems ineffective against more serious infections, such as **infectious mononucleosis, measles, typhoid fever, tuberculosis, syphilis,** and the like.

Owing to restricted bile flow in the liver and gallbladder, the small intestine is restricted in its capacity to digest food properly. This permits substantial amounts of waste matter and poisonous substances, such as *cadaverines* and *putrescines* (breakdown products of putrefied food), to seep into the lymphatic ducts. These toxins, along with fats and proteins, enter the body's largest lymph vessel, the *thoracic duct,* at the *cysterna chyli.* The cysterna chyli are dilated lymph vessels in the shape of sacks, situated in front of the first two lumbar vertebrae (see **Figure 9**) at the level of the belly button.

Toxins, antigens, and undigested proteins from animal sources, including fish, meat, eggs, and dairy foods, as well as leaked plasma proteins, cause these lymph sacks to swell and become inflamed. When the cells of an animal become damaged or die, which happens seconds after it is killed, its protein structures are broken down by cellular enzymes. These so-called "degenerate" proteins are useless for the body, and they become harmful unless they are promptly removed by the lymphatic system. Their presence usually invites enhanced microbial activity. Viruses, fungi, and bacteria feed on the pooled wastes. In some cases, allergic reactions occur.

When the cysterna chyli (lymph sacks) are overtaxed and congested, the lymphatic system is no longer able to sufficiently remove even the body's own degenerate proteins (from worn-out cells). This results in **lymph edema.** While lying on the back, existing lymph edema can be felt as hard knots, sometimes as large as a fist, in the area of the belly button. These "rocks" are a major cause of **middle and low back pain** and **abdominal swelling,** and, in fact, of most symptoms of ill health. Many people who have grown a "tummy" consider this abdominal extension to be just a harmless nuisance or a natural part of aging. They don't realize that they are breeding a living "time bomb" that may go off some day and injure vital parts of the body. Anyone with a bloated abdomen suffers from major lymph congestion.

Some 80 percent of the lymphatic system is associated with the intestines, making this area of the body the largest center of immune activity. This is no coincidence. The part of the body where most disease-causing agents are combated or generated is, in fact, the intestinal tract. Any lymph edema, or other kind of obstruction in this important part of the lymphatic system, can lead to potentially serious complications elsewhere in the body.

Wherever a lymph duct is obstructed, lymph has also accumulated at some distance from the obstruction. Consequently, the lymph nodes located in such an area can no longer adequately neutralize or detoxify the following things: dead and live phagocytes and their ingested microbes, worn-out tissue cells, cells damaged by disease, products of fermentation, pesticides in food, toxic antibodies contained in most plant foods, inhaled or otherwise ingested chemical particles, cells from malignant tumors, and the millions of cancer cells every healthy person generates each day. Incomplete destruction of these things can cause these lymph nodes to become inflamed, enlarged, and congested with blood. Infected material may enter the bloodstream, causing septic poisoning and acute illnesses. In most cases, though, the lymph blockage occurs slowly, without any symptoms other than swelling of the abdomen, hands, arms, feet, or ankles, or sometimes puffiness in the face and eyes. This is often referred to as "water retention," a major precursor of chronic illness.

Continuous lymphatic obstruction usually leads to chronic health problems. Almost every chronic illness results from congestion in the cysterna chyli. Eventually, the thoracic duct, which drains the cysterna chyli, is overburdened by the constant influx of toxic material and becomes clogged up, too. The thoracic duct is linked with numerous other lymph ducts (see **Figures 9 and 10**) that empty their waste into the thoracic "sewer canal."

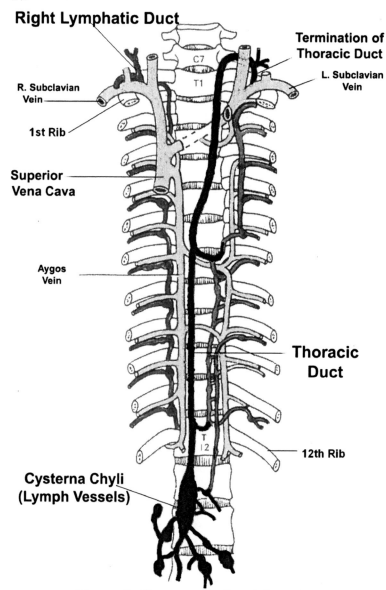

Figure 9: Cysterna chyli and thoracic duct

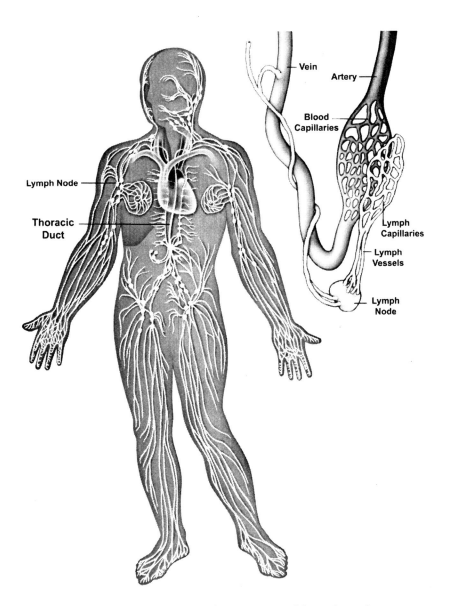

Figure 10: Lymphatic system and lymph node

Since the thoracic duct has to remove nearly 85 percent of the body's daily-generated cellular waste and other potentially hazardous material, a blockage there causes backing up of waste into other, more distant parts of the body.

When the daily-generated metabolic waste and cellular debris are not removed from an area in the body for a certain length of time, symptoms of disease start to manifest. The following are but a few typical examples of illness indicators that result directly from chronic, localized lymph congestion:

Obesity, cysts in the uterus or ovaries, enlargement of the prostate gland, rheumatism in the joints, enlargement of the left half of the heart, congestive heart failure, congested bronchi and lungs, swelling or enlargement of the neck area, stiffness in the neck and shoulders, backaches, headaches, migraines, dizziness, vertigo, ringing in the ears, earaches, deafness, dandruff, frequent colds, sinusitis, hay fever, certain types of asthma, thyroid enlargement, eye diseases, poor vision, swelling in the breasts, breast cancer, kidney problems, lower back pains, swelling of the legs and ankles, scoliosis, brain disorders, memory loss, stomach trouble, enlarged spleen, irritable bowel syndrome, hernia, polyps in the colon, and others.

The thoracic duct typically empties its detoxified waste contents into the left *subclavian vein* at the root of the neck. This vein enters the *superior vena cava,* which leads straight into the heart. In addition to blocking proper lymph drainage from the various organs or parts of the body, congestion in the cysterna chyli and thoracic duct permits toxic materials to be passed into the heart and heart arteries. This unduly stresses the heart. It also allows these toxins and disease-causing agents to enter the general circulation and spread to other parts of the body. Hardly a disease can be named that is not caused by lymphatic obstruction. Lymph blockage, in most cases, has its origin in a congested liver (the causes of gallstones in the liver will be discussed in the following chapter). In the extreme eventuality, **lymphoma** or **cancer of the lymph** may result, of which **Hodgkin's disease** is the most common type.

When the circulatory system begins to malfunction because of gallstones in the liver, the *endocrine system* starts to be affected as well. The endocrine glands produce hormones that pass directly from the glandular cells into the bloodstream, where they influence bodily activity, growth, and nutrition. The glands most often affected by congestion are the thyroid, parathyroid, adrenal cortex, ovaries, and testes. A more severely disrupted circulatory function leads to imbalanced hormone secretions by the *islets of Langerhans* in the pancreas and the *pineal* and *pituitary glands.* Blood congestion, which is characterized by the thickening of the blood, prevents hormones from reaching their target places in the body in sufficient amounts and on time. Consequently, the glands go into *hypersecretion* (overproduction) of hormones.

When lymph drainage from the glands is inefficient, the glands themselves become congested. This brings about *hyposecretion* (lack) of hormones. Diseases related to imbalances of the thyroid gland include **toxic goiter, Graves' disease, cretinism, myxoedema, tumors of the thyroid, hypoparathyroidism. Thyroid disorders can also** reduce calcium absorption and cause **cataracts,** as well as **behavioral disorders** and **dementia.** Poor calcium absorption, alone, is responsible for numerous diseases, including **osteoporosis** (loss of bone density). If circulatory problems disrupt the secretion of balanced amounts of insulin in the pancreatic islets of Langerhans, **diabetes** may develop.

Gallstones in the liver can cause liver cells to cut down protein synthesis. Reduced protein synthesis, in turn, prompts the adrenal glands to overproduce *cortisol,* a hormone that stimulates protein synthesis. Too much *cortisol* in the blood gives rise to **atrophy of lymphoid tissue** and a **depressed immune response,** which is considered the leading cause of cancer and many other major illnesses.

An imbalance in the secretion of adrenal hormones can cause a wide variety of disorders, as it leads to weakened **febrile response** (fever) and **diminished protein synthesis.** Proteins are the major building blocks for tissue cells, hormones, and so forth. The liver is capable of producing many different hormones. Hormones determine how well the body grows and heals.

The liver also inhibits certain hormones, including *insulin, glucagon, cortisol, aldosterone, thyroid,* and *sex hormones.* Gallstones in the liver impair this vital function, which may increase hormone concentrations in the blood. Hormone imbalance is an extremely serious condition and can easily occur when gallstones in the liver have disrupted major circulatory pathways that are also hormonal pathways. For example, by failing to keep blood cortisol levels balanced, a person may accumulate excessive amounts of fat in the body. If estrogens are not broken down properly, the risk of breast cancer increases. If blood insulin is not broken down properly, the risk of cancer rises, and the cells in the body may become resistant to insulin, which is a major precursor of diabetes.

Disease is naturally absent when blood flow and lymph flow are both unhindered and normal. Both types of problems—circulatory and lymphatic—can be successfully eliminated through a series of liver flushes and prevented by following a balanced diet and lifestyle.

Disorders of the Respiratory System

Both mental and physical health depend on the effectiveness and vitality of the cells in the body. The cells of the body derive most of their energy from chemical reactions that take place in the presence of oxygen. One of the resultant waste products is carbon dioxide. The respiratory system provides the routes by which oxygen is taken into the body and carbon dioxide is excreted. Blood serves as the transport system for the exchange of these gases between the lungs and the cells.

Gallstones in the liver can impair respiratory functions and cause **allergies, disorders of the nose and nasal cavities**, and **diseases of the bronchi and lungs.** When gallstones distort or injure the lobules (units) of the liver, the blood-cleansing ability of the liver, small intestine, lymphatic system, and immune system diminishes. Waste material and toxic substances, normally rendered harmless by these organs and systems, now begin to seep into the heart, lungs, bronchi, and other respiratory passages. Constant exposure to these irritating agents lowers the resistance of the respiratory system to them. Lymph congestion in the abdominal region, particularly in the cysterna chyli and thoracic duct, hampers proper lymphatic drainage from the respiratory organs. Most respiratory ailments occur because of such lymph blockages.

Pneumonia results when protective measures fail to prevent inhaled or blood-borne microbes from reaching and colonizing the lungs. Gallstones harbor harmful microbes, as well as highly toxic, irritating material that can enter the blood via areas in the liver that are damaged by the presence of gallstones. Gallstones are a constant source of immune suppression, which leaves the body, and particularly the upper respiratory tract, susceptible to both internal and external disease-triggering factors. These include both blood-borne and airborne microbes (believed to cause pneumonia), cigarette smoke, alcohol, x-rays, corticosteroids, allergens, antigens, common pollutants, waste matter from the GI tract, and the like.

Further respiratory complications arise when handfuls of gallstones that have accumulated in the liver bile ducts lead to **liver enlargement.** The liver, situated in the upper abdominal cavity, spans almost the entire width of the body. Its upper and anterior surfaces are smooth and shaped to fit under the surface of the diaphragm. When enlarged, the liver obstructs the movement of the diaphragm and prevents the lungs from extending to their normal capacity during inhalation. By contrast, a smooth, healthy liver permits the lungs to easily extend into the abdominal region, which puts pressure on the abdomen and squeezes the lymph and blood vessels to force lymph and blood toward the heart. This breathing mechanism is often called "belly breathing," and it can be seen in healthy babies, especially. An enlarged liver prevents the full extension of the diaphragm and lungs, which causes reduced exchange of gases in the lungs, lymphatic congestion, and the retention of excessive amounts of carbon dioxide in the lungs. The restricted uptake of oxygen negatively affects cellular functions throughout the body.

Most people in the industrialized world have an enlarged liver, especially those who are overweight or obese. What doctors generally consider a "normal-sized" liver is actually oversize. Once all gallstones are removed through a series of liver flushes, the liver can gradually return to its original size.

Almost all diseases of the lungs, bronchi, and upper respiratory passages are either caused or worsened by gallstones in the liver and can be improved or eliminated by removing these stones through liver cleansing.

Disorders of the Urinary System

The *urinary system* is an extremely important excretory system of the body. It consists of the following: two *kidneys,* which form and excrete urine; two *ureters,* which convey the urine from the kidneys to the urinary bladder; a *urinary bladder,* where urine collects and is temporarily stored; and a *urethra,* through which urine passes from the urinary bladder to the exterior of the body (see **Figure 11**).

Smooth functioning of the urinary system is essential for maintaining an appropriate fluid volume by regulating the amount of water that is excreted in the urine. Other aspects of its function include regulating the concentrations of various electrolytes in the body fluids and maintaining normal pH (acids-alkalis balance) of the blood. This system is also involved in the disposal of waste products resulting from the breakdown (catabolism) of cell protein in the liver, for example.

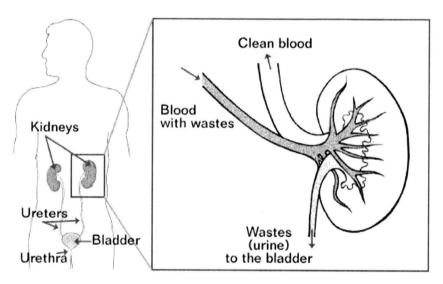

Figure 11: The urinary system

Most diseases of the kidneys and other parts of the urinary system are related to an imbalance of the *simple filtration* system in the kidneys. About 26 to 40 gallons of dilute filtrate are formed each day by the two kidneys. Of these, only 34 to 52 ounces are excreted as urine (the rest is absorbed and recirculated). With the exception of blood cells, platelets, and blood proteins, all other blood constituents must pass through the kidneys. The process of filtration is disrupted and weakened when the digestive system—and. in particular, the liver—perform poorly.

Gallstones in the liver and gallbladder reduce the amount of bile that the liver is able to produce. Thus, it becomes impossible to digest food properly. Much of the undigested food begins to ferment and putrefy, leaving toxic waste matter in the blood and lymph. The body's normal excretions, such as urine, sweat, gases, and feces, do not usually contain disease-generating waste products; that is, of course, for as long as the passages of elimination remain clear and unobstructed.

Disease-causing agents consist of tiny molecules that appear in the blood and lymph. They are visible only through powerful electron microscopes. These molecules have a strong acidifying effect on the blood. To avoid a life-threatening disease or coma, the blood must rid itself of these minute toxins. Accordingly, it dumps these unwanted intruders into the connective tissue of the organs. The connective tissue consists of a gel-like fluid (lymph) that surrounds all cells. The cells are "bathed" in this connective tissue. Under normal circumstances, the body knows how to deal with acidic waste material that has been dumped into the connective tissue. It releases an alkaline product, *sodium bicarbonate* ($NaHCO_3$) into the blood that is able to retrieve the acidic toxins, neutralize them, and then eliminate them through the excretory organs. This emergency system, though, begins to fail when toxins are deposited faster than they can be retrieved and eliminated. As a result, the connective tissue may become as thick as jelly. Nutrients, water, and oxygen can no longer pass freely, and the cells of the organs begin to suffer malnutrition, dehydration, and oxygen deficiency.

Some of the most acidic compounds are proteins from animal foods. Gallstones inhibit the liver's ability to break down these proteins. Excessive proteins are "temporarily" stored in the connective tissues and then converted into collagen fiber. The collagen fiber is built into the basal membranes of the capillary walls. The basal membranes may become up to ten times as thick as normal. A similar situation occurs in the arteries. As the blood vessel walls become increasingly congested, fewer proteins are able to escape the bloodstream. This leads to blood thickening, making it more and more difficult for the kidneys to filter. At the same time, the basal membranes of the blood vessels supplying the kidneys also become congested, making them harder and more rigid. As the process of hardening of the blood vessels progresses further, **blood pressure** starts to rise and overall kidney performance drops. More and more of the metabolic waste products excreted by the kidney cells, which would normally be eliminated via venous blood vessels and lymphatic ducts, are now retained and adversely affect the performance of the kidneys even further.

Through all this, the kidneys become overburdened and can no longer maintain normal fluid and electrolyte balances in the body. In addition, urinary components may precipitate and form into crystals and stones of various types and sizes (see **Figure 12a**). **Uric acid stones,** for example, are formed when uric acid concentration in the urine exceeds 2 to 4 mg percent. This amount was considered within the range of tolerance until the mid-1960s, when it was adjusted upward. Uric acid is a by-product of the breakdown of protein in the liver. Since meat consumption rose sharply in that decade, the "within the norm" level was adjusted to 7.5 mg percent. This adjustment, however, does not make uric acid any less harmful to the body. Stones formed from excessive uric acid concentrations of 4 mg percent and higher (also see "Bladder stones" in **Figure 12b**) can lead to **urinary obstruction, kidney infection,** and, eventually, **kidney failure.**

As kidney cells become increasingly deprived of vital nutrients, including oxygen, malignant tumors may develop. In addition, uric acid crystals that are not eliminated by the kidneys can settle in the joints and cause rheumatism, gout, and water retention.

Symptoms of impending kidney trouble are often deceptively mild in comparison to the potential severity of kidney disease. The most observable and common symptoms of kidney problems are abnormal changes in the volume, frequency, and coloration of the urine. These are usually accompanied by swelling of the eyes, face, and ankles, as well as pain in the upper and lower back. If the disease has progressed further, there may be blurred vision, tiredness, declined performance, and nausea. The following symptoms may also indicate malfunctioning of the kidneys: *high blood pressure, low blood pressure, pain moving from the upper to lower abdomen, dark-brown urine, pain in the back just above the waist, excessive thirst, increase in urination (especially during the night), less than 500 ml of urine per day, a feeling of fullness in the bladder, pain while passing urine, drier and browner skin pigment, ankles being puffy at night, eyes being puffy in morning, bruising, and hemorrhaging.*

All major diseases of the urinary system are caused by toxic blood; in other words, by blood filled with tiny molecules of waste material and excessive proteins. Gallstones in the liver impair digestion, cause blood and lymph congestion, and disrupt the entire circulatory system, including that of the urinary system.

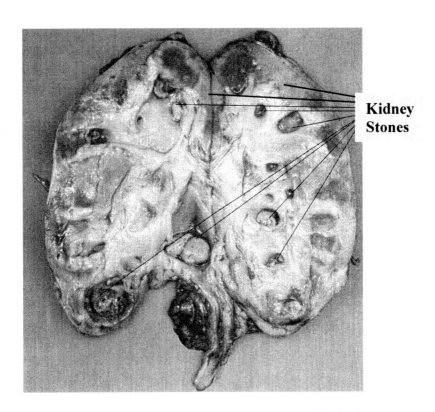

Kidney Stones

Figure 12a: Kidney stones embedded in kidney

49

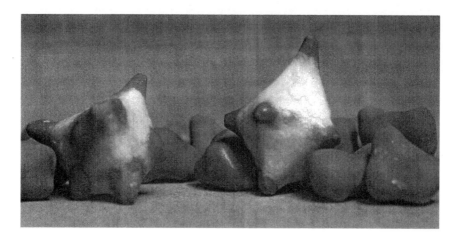

Figure 12b: Bladder stones

When the gallstones are removed, the urinary system has a chance to recuperate, rid itself of accumulated toxins and stones, and maintain fluid balance and normal blood pressure. This is necessary for all the processes in the body to run smoothly and efficiently. There may also be a strong need to cleanse the kidneys, in addition to the liver and gallbladder (see *The Kidney Cleanse,* section 3 of Chapter 5).

Disorders of the Nervous System

Our entire lives are dictated by the way we feel. Our persona, the way we carry ourselves, our interactions with other people, our moods, cravings, patience and tolerance levels, and our reactions to life's occurrences—all are strongly influenced by the condition of our nervous system. In today's fast-paced world, we are exposed to a variety of conditions that wreak havoc on our bodies. The brain is the control center of the body, and unless it receives proper nourishment, your entire physical and emotional being can easily become chaotic.

Brain cells are normally easily capable of manufacturing the huge number of chemicals they need for the complex tasks they must perform, day after day, year after year. However, their life support depends on the continuous supply of nutrients necessary to produce those chemicals. Modern intensive agriculture has nearly depleted farm soil of all its basic nutrients (see *Take Ionic Essential Minerals,* section 5 in Chapter 5). Although this has certainly added to the nutritional deficiencies so prevalent among the populations in industrialized nations, most nutrient deficiencies actually occur as a result of poor performance of the digestive system and, particularly, of the liver. Lack of such nutrients can hinder the ability of our brains to manufacture the chemicals they need to function efficiently.

The brain can operate for quite some time with substandard amounts of nutrients, but the price one pays includes poor health, fatigue, lack of energy, mood swings, depression, sickness, aches and pains, and general discomfort. Some deficiencies manifest in mental disease, such as schizophrenia and Alzheimer's.

The health of the nervous system, which includes the brain, the spinal cord, pairs of spinal and cranial nerves, and autonomic functions, largely depends on the quality of the blood. Blood is composed of plasma (a straw-colored transparent fluid) and cells. The constituents of plasma are water, plasma proteins, mineral salts, hormones, vitamins, nutrient materials, organic waste products, antibodies, and gases. There are three varieties of blood cells: white cells (*leukocytes*), red cells (*erythrocytes*), and platelets (*thrombocytes*). Any abnormal changes in the blood affect the nervous system as well as the rest of the body.

All three types of blood cells are formed in the red bone marrow, which is nourished and maintained by the nutrients supplied by the digestive system. Gallstones in the liver interfere with the digestion and assimilation of food, which fills the plasma of the blood with excessive waste material and reduces nutrient supplies to the red bone marrow. This, in turn, upsets the balance of blood cell constituents, disrupts hormonal pathways, and causes abnormal responses in the nervous system. Most diseases afflicting the nervous system are rooted in improperly formed blood, brought about by a dysfunctional liver and subsequent waste accumulation in the intestinal tract.

Each of the numerous functions of the liver has a direct influence on the nervous system, particularly the brain. The liver cells convert glycogen (complex sugar) into glucose, which, besides oxygen and water, serves as the most important nutrient for the nervous system. Glucose covers most of that system's energy requirements.

The brain, although it constitutes only one-fiftieth of the body's weight, contains about one-fifth of the total blood volume in the body. It uses up vast amounts of glucose. Gallstones in the liver drastically reduce glucose supplies to the brain and the rest of the nervous system. This, in turn, can affect the performance of the organs, senses, and mind. At the early stages of imbalance, a person may develop food cravings, particularly for sweet or starchy foods, and experience frequent mood swings or emotional stress.

There are other, even more serious problems arising from occurrence of gallstones in the liver. The liver forms the plasma proteins and most of the blood-clotting factors from the body's amino acid pool. Occurrence of gallstones in the bile ducts of the liver increasingly inhibits this important function. When the production of clotting factors drops, platelet count drops, too, and there may be spontaneous capillary bleeding or **hemorrhagic disease.** If a hemorrhage occurs in the brain, it may cause destruction of brain tissue, paralysis, or death. The severity of the bleeding may be determined by such variable triggers as hypertension and alcohol abuse. Platelet counts also drop when the production of new cells does not keep pace with the destruction of damaged or worn-out cells; this occurs when gallstones cut off the blood supply to the liver cells.

Vitamin K is another element essential for the synthesis of major clotting factors. It is a fat-soluble vitamin stored in the liver. To absorb fats in the intestines, the body requires bile salts that are made available through bile secretions. Gallstones in the liver and gallbladder obstruct bile flow, which leads to inadequate fat absorption and subsequent vitamin K deficiency.

As discussed earlier, gallstones in the liver can lead to disorders of the vascular system. When the blood undergoes changes and becomes too thick, blood vessels begin to harden and become damaged. If a blood clot forms in an injured artery, a piece of that blood clot (*embolus*) may lodge in a small artery distant from the injury and obstruct the blood flow, causing **ischemia** and **infarction.** If the infarction occurs in a brain artery, it is called a **stroke.**

All circulatory disturbances affect the brain and the rest of the nervous system. The disruption of liver functions particularly affects *astrocytes*—cells that form the main supporting tissue of the central nervous system. This condition is characterized by apathy, disorientation, brain fog, delirium, muscular rigidity, and coma. Nitrogenous bacterial waste absorbed from the colon, unless detoxified by the liver, may reach the brain cells via the blood. Other metabolic waste products, such as ammonia, may reach toxic concentrations and change the permeability of the blood vessels in the brain, thus reducing the effectiveness of the blood-brain barrier. This may permit various noxious substances to enter the brain and cause further damage. If a large number of neurons of the brain no longer receive enough nourishment, there is atrophy of neural tissue, which leads to **dementia** or **Alzheimer's disease.** When a certain class of neurons that are responsible for producing the brain hormone and neurotransmitter *dopamine* suffer malnourishment, **Parkinson's disease** results. Repeated exposure to certain environmental or internally produced toxins can also be responsible.

Multiple sclerosis (MS) occurs when the cells that produce *myelin* (a sheath of fatty material that surrounds most axons of nerve cells) suffer malnutrition and insufficient lymph drainage. The myelin sheath diminishes, and axons become injured. MS patients always suffer from progressive congestion in the large intestine; this prevents proper nutrient absorption. Cleansing the eliminative organs and improving nutrition are among the most powerful approaches to halt and possibly reverse MS.

The liver controls the digestion, absorption, and metabolism of fatty substances throughout the body. Gallstones interfere with fat metabolism and affect cholesterol levels in the blood. *Cholesterol* is an essential building block of all our body cells and is needed for every metabolic process. Our brains consist of more than 10 percent pure cholesterol (all water removed). Cholesterol is important for brain development and brain function. It protects the nerves against damage or injury. An imbalance of blood fats can profoundly affect the nervous system and, thereby, cause almost any type of illness in the body. Removing gallstones from the liver and gallbladder increases nutrient supplies to all the cells, thus rejuvenating the nervous system and improving all functions in the body.

Disorders of the Bone

Although bone is the hardest tissue in the body, it is, nevertheless, very much alive. Human bone consists of 20 percent water; 30–40 percent organic material, such as living cells; and 40–50 percent inorganic material, such as calcium. Bone tissue contains many blood and lymph vessels and nerves. The cells responsible for balanced bone growth are *osteoblasts* and *osteoclasts*. Osteoblasts are the bone-forming cells, whereas osteoclasts are responsible for resorption of bone to maintain optimum shape. A third group of cells, known as *chondrocytes,* are in charge of forming cartilage. The less dense parts of the bone, called *cancellous bone,* contain red bone marrow, which produces red and white blood cells.

Most bone diseases occur when bone cells no longer receive enough nourishment. Gallstones in the liver usually lead to lymph congestion in the intestinal tract and, consequently, in other parts of the body (see *Disorders of the Circulatory System*). Good bone health results from the sustained balance between the functions of osteoblast and osteoclast cells. This delicate balance becomes disturbed when nutrient supply is deficient and thereby slows the production of new bone tissue by osteoblasts. **Osteoporosis** results when the amount of bone tissue is reduced because the growth of new bone does not keep pace with the destruction of old bone. *Cancellous* bone is usually affected before *compact bone* is. Compact bone makes up the outer layer of the bone.

In generalized osteoporosis, excessive calcium is reabsorbed from bone, thereby raising the calcium levels of blood and urine. This may predispose a person to form stones in the kidneys and, possibly, suffer renal failure. Gallstones in the liver substantially reduce bile production. Bile is essential for the absorption of calcium from the small intestines. Even if the body received more than enough calcium foods or food supplements, a shortage of bile would render much of the ingested calcium useless for bone building and other important metabolic processes. In addition, the presence of gallstones in the liver raises the level of harmful acids in the blood, some of which are neutralized by calcium leached from the bones and teeth. (Something similar happens when a person drinks cow's milk. To neutralize the high phosphorus concentration of ingested milk, the body uses not only the milk's calcium but also calcium from the bones and teeth.)

Eventually, the body's calcium reserves become depleted, diminishing bone density or bone mass. This may lead to bone and hip fractures and even death. With more than half of all women over age 50 already affected by osteoporosis (albeit only in industrialized nations), it is obvious that the current approach of taking hormones or calcium supplements is a shot in the dark; it in no way addresses the imbalance in the liver and gallbladder caused by reduced bile output due to gallstones.

Rickets and **osteomalacia** are diseases that affect the calcification process of bones. In either case, the bones become soft, especially those of the lower limbs, which are *bowed* by the weight of the body. The fat-soluble vitamin D, *calciferol,* is essential for balanced calcium and phosphorus metabolism and, therefore, healthy bone structures. Insufficient bile secretion and disturbance of the cholesterol metabolism, both of which are caused by gallstones in the liver, lead to vitamin D deficiency. Lack of sufficient exposure to natural sunlight further aggravates these conditions.

Infection of bones, or **osteomyelitis,** may result when there has been a prolonged lymphatic obstruction in the body, especially in or around bone tissues. Consequently, blood-borne microbes gain unhindered access to bones. As mentioned before, infectious microbes only attack tissues that are acidified, weak, unstable, or damaged. The microbes may originate from gallstones, a tooth abscess, or a boil.

Malignant tumors of the bone can occur when lymphatic congestion in the body and the bones, especially, has reached extreme proportions. The immune system is depressed, and malignant tumor particles from the breasts, lungs, or prostate gland can spread to or develop in those parts of the bones that have the softest tissue and are more prone to congestion and acidification, that is, the cancellous bone. Bone cancer and all other diseases of the bone indicate lack of nourishment of bone tissue. Such diseases usually defy treatment unless all gallstones in the liver are removed and all other organs and systems of elimination are cleared of any existing congestion as well.

Disorders of the Joints

Our body contains three types of joints: *fibrous* or fib joints, *cartilaginous* or slightly movable joints, and *synovial* or freely movable joints. The most susceptible to disease are the joints of the hands, feet, knees, shoulders, elbows, and hips. **Rheumatoid arthritis, osteoarthritis,** and **gout** are among the most commonly found joint disorders.

Most people stricken with rheumatoid arthritis have a long history of intestinal complaints: **bloating, flatulence, heartburn, belching, constipation, diarrhea, coldness and swelling of hands and feet, increased perspiration, general fatigue, loss of appetite, weight reduction, and more.** It is reasonable, therefore, to conclude that rheumatoid arthritis is linked with any of these, or similar, symptoms of major intestinal and metabolic disturbances. I have personally experienced all the symptoms mentioned above when I suffered painful bouts of juvenile rheumatoid arthritis during my childhood years.

The GI tract is constantly exposed to a large number of viruses, bacteria, and parasites. In addition to the many *antigens* (foreign materials) contained in foods, the digestive system may also have to deal with insecticides, pesticides, hormones, antibiotic residues, preservatives, and colorings contained in so many foodstuffs today, as well as some large-molecule drugs such as penicillin. Possible antigens include pollen from flowers, plants, plant antibodies, fungi, bacteria, and the like. It is the task of the immune system, most of which is located in the intestinal wall, to protect us against all these potentially harmful invaders and substances. To be able to accomplish this task every day, both the digestive and lymphatic systems must remain unobstructed and efficient. Gallstones in the liver seriously disturb the digestive process, which leads to an overload of toxic substances in the blood and lymph, as mentioned above (see *Disorders of the Circulatory System*).

Doctors consider *arthritis* an *autoimmune disease* affecting the synovial membrane. Autoimmunity, a condition in which the immune system develops immunity to its own cells, results when antigen/antibody complexes (*rheumatoid factors*) are formed in the blood. Naturally, the B-lymphocytes (immune cells) in the intestinal wall become stimulated and produce antibodies (*immunoglobulins*) when coming into contact with these antigens. The immune cells circulate in the blood, and some settle in the lymph nodes, spleen, mucus membranes of the salivary glands, lymphatic system of the bronchial tubes, vagina or uterus, milk-producing mammary glands of the breasts, and capsular tissues of the joints.

If there is repeated exposure to the same types of toxic antigens, antibody production will increase dramatically, particularly in areas where immune cells have settled because of a previous encounter with the invaders. These harmful antigens may consist of protein particles from putrefying animal foods, for example. In such a case, intense microbial activity can occur. The new encounter with the antigens raises the level of antigen/antibody complexes in the blood and upsets the fine balance that exists between the immune reaction and its suppression. Autoimmune diseases, which indicate an extremely high level of toxicity in the body, directly result from a disturbance of this balance. If antibody production is continually high in synovial joints, inflammation becomes chronic, leading to gradually increasing deformity, pain, and loss of function.

The overuse of the immune system leads to *self-destruction* in the body. If this form of self-destruction occurs in nerve tissue, it is called MS, and if it occurs in organ tissue, it is called cancer. Yet, seen from a deeper perspective, the self-destruction is but a final attempt at self-preservation. The body only "attacks" itself if the toxicity has increased to such a degree that it could cause more damage than an autoimmune response would. It certainly has no intention of committing suicide, which is what the meaning of "autoimmune disease" suggests. When the body's cell membranes are clogged with foreign, harmful chemicals and toxic particles like trans fatty acids (as found in fast foods, such as hamburgers and French fries), it is an absolutely normal response by the immune system to attack these contaminants. To call this survival response a disease is unscientific and reflects a lack of knowledge of the true nature of the body.

Gallstones inhibit the body's ability to keep itself nourished and clean, which makes them a leading cause of toxicity. They prevent the liver from adequately taking noxious substances out of the bloodstream. If the liver cannot filter out toxins from the blood, they end up being dumped into the extracellular fluid. The more toxins accumulate in the extracellular fluid, the more severely that cell membranes become clogged with injurious materials. An autoimmune response may be necessary to destroy the most contaminated cells and thereby save the rest of the body, at least for a while. When all gallstones are removed from the liver and gallbladder, the immune system does not have to take recourse to such extreme measures of defending the body on the cellular level.

Osteoarthritis is a degenerative, noninflammatory illness. It occurs when the renewal of *articular cartilage* (a smooth, strong surface, covering bones that are in contact with other bones) does not keep pace with its removal. The articular cartilage gradually becomes thinner until, eventually, the bony articular surfaces come into contact, and the bones begin to degenerate. Abnormal bone repair and chronic inflammation may follow this form of damage. Like most diseases, this symptom results from a long-standing digestive disorder. As fewer nutrients are absorbed and distributed for tissue building, it becomes increasingly difficult to maintain healthy sustenance of bone and articular cartilage. Gallstones in the liver impair the basic digestive processes and, therefore, play perhaps the most important role in the development of osteoarthritis.

Gout, which is another joint disease connected to weak liver performance, is caused by *sodium urate crystals* in joints and tendons. Gout occurs in some people whose *blood uric acid* is abnormally high. When gallstones in the liver begin to affect blood circulation in the kidneys (see *Disorders of the Urinary System*), uric acid excretion becomes inefficient. This also causes increased cell damage and cell destruction in the liver and kidneys, as well as in other parts of the body.

Uric acid is a waste product resulting from the breakdown of cell nuclei; it is produced in excess with increased cell destruction. Smoking cigarettes, drinking alcoholic beverages regularly, using stimulants, and so forth, all cause marked cell destruction, which releases large quantities of degenerate cell protein into the bloodstream. In addition, uric acid production rises sharply with overconsumption of protein foods, such as meat, fish, pork, and eggs.[12] Incidentally, all the aforementioned foods and substances lead to gallstone formation in the liver and gallbladder.

A person may experience several acute attacks of arthritis before damage to the joints decreases mobility and the gout condition becomes chronic.

Disorders of the Reproductive System

Female and male reproductive systems both depend largely on the smooth functioning of the liver. Gallstones in the liver obstruct the movement of bile through the bile ducts, which impairs digestion and distorts the structural framework of liver lobules. This diminishes the liver's production of both *serum albumin* and *clotting factors.* Serum albumin is the most common and abundant protein in the blood, responsible for maintaining *plasma osmotic pressure* at its normal level of 25mmHg. *Clotting factors* are essential for the coagulation of blood. Insufficient osmotic pressure cuts down the supply of nutrients to the cells, including those of the reproductive organs. This may lead to reduced lymph drainage. Poor lymph drainage from the reproductive organs can cause fluid retention and edema, as well as the retention of metabolic waste and dead cells. All of this may result in the gradual impairment of sexual functions.

Most diseases of the reproductive system result from improper lymph drainage. The thoracic duct (see *Disorders of the Circulatory System*) drains lymph fluid from all organs of the digestive system, including the liver, spleen, pancreas, stomach, and intestines. This large duct often becomes severely congested when gallstones in the liver impair proper digestion and absorption of food. It is obvious, yet hardly recognized in mainstream medicine, that congestion in the thoracic duct affects the organs of

---

[12] Also see "The Kidney Cleanse" in the book *Timeless Secrets of Health and Rejuvenation* by the author.

the reproductive system. These organs, like most others in the body, need to release their turned-over cells and metabolic waste matter into the thoracic duct.

Impaired lymphatic drainage from the female pelvic area is responsible for **suppressed immunity, menstrual problems, premenstrual stress (PMS), menopausal symptoms, pelvic inflammatory disease (PID), cervicitis, all uterine diseases, vulvar dystrophies with growth of fibrous tissue, ovarian cysts and tumors, cell destruction, hormone deficiencies, low libido, infertility, and genetic mutations of cells leading to cancer.**

Thoracic blockage may also lead to lymph congestion in the left breast, thereby leaving deposits of noxious substances behind that can cause inflammation, lump formation, milk duct blockage, and cancerous tumors. If the right lymphatic duct, which drains lymph from the right half of the thorax, head, neck, and right arm, becomes congested, waste accumulates in the right breast, leading to similar problems there.

A continuous restriction of lymph drainage from the male pelvic area causes benign and malignant prostate enlargement as well as inflammation of the testes, penis, and urethra. Impotence is a likely consequence of this development. The consistent increase of gallstones in the liver, a common factor among middle-aged men in affluent societies, is one of the major reasons for lymph blockage in this vital part of the body. Venereal diseases occur when the exposed parts of the body reach a high level of toxicity. Microbial infection is preceded by major lymph congestion. The collapsing capacity of the lymphatic system (which includes the immune system) to repel invading microorganisms is the true reason for most reproductive and sexual disorders.

When all gallstones from the liver are removed and a healthy diet and lifestyle are maintained, lymphatic activity can return to normal. The reproductive tissue receives improved nourishment and becomes more resistant. Infections subside; cysts, fibrous tissue, and tumors are broken down and removed; and sexual functions are restored.

Disorders of the Skin

Nearly all skin diseases such as **eczema, acne,** and **psoriasis** have one factor in common: gallstones in the liver. Almost every person with a skin disease also has intestinal problems and impure blood, in particular. These are mainly caused by gallstones and the harmful effects they have on the body as a whole. Gallstones contribute to numerous problems throughout the body—particularly in the digestive, circulatory, and urinary systems. In its attempt to eliminate what the colon, kidneys, lungs, liver, and lymphatic system are unable to remove or detoxify, the skin becomes flooded and overburdened with acidic waste. Although the skin is the largest organ of elimination in the body, it eventually succumbs to the acid assault. The toxic material is deposited first in the connective tissue underneath the *dermis*. When this "waste depot" becomes saturated, the skin begins to malfunction.

Excessive amounts of noxious substances, cell debris, microbes from different sources (such as gallstones), and various antigens from improperly digested foods congest the lymphatic system and inhibit proper lymph drainage from the various, living layers of the skin. The toxins and putrefying protein from damaged or destroyed skin cells attract microbes and become a source of constant irritation and inflammation of the skin. Skin cells begin to suffer malnourishment, which may greatly reduce their normal interval of turnover (about once every month). This may also cause extensive damage to skin nerves.

If the sebaceous glands, which pour their secretion, *sebum,* into the hair follicles, become nutrient deficient, hair growth becomes abnormal and, in particular, **scalp hair may fall out.** When the body's *melanin* supply becomes deficient, the **hair turns gray** prematurely. Sebum deficiency alters the healthy texture of the hair and makes it look dull and unattractive. On the skin, sebum acts as a bactericidal and fungicidal agent, preventing the invasion of microbes. It also prevents drying and cracking of the skin, especially when exposed to sunshine and hot, dry air.

A genetic predisposition toward developing baldness or any other skin disorder may play a role but is *not* a major causative factor, as is often assumed. Healthy skin functions are often completely restored and hair growth, particularly among women, is returned to normal once all gallstones are removed and the colon and kidneys/bladder are kept clean. (For details regarding colonic irrigation and kidney cleansing, refer to my book, *Timeless Secrets of Health and Rejuvenation.*)

Conclusion

Gallstones are a major cause of illness in the body. They impair the functioning of one of the more complex, active, and influential organs of the body—the liver. Nobody has ever devised an artificial liver, because it is so complex. Second only to the brain in complexity, the liver masterminds the most intricate processes of digestion and metabolism, thereby affecting the life and health of every cell in the body. When a person removes the obstacles that prevent the liver from doing its job properly and efficiently, his or her body can return to a state of continuous balance and vitality.

Chapter 2

How Can I Tell I Have Gallstones?

During my research with thousands of patients suffering from almost every kind of illness, including *terminal diseases*, I found that each person had large numbers of gallstones in the liver and, in many cases, also in the gallbladder. When these people eliminated these stones through the liver flush and introduced simple health-forming habits and supportive measures, they recovered from diseases that defied both conventional and alternative methods of treatment.

What follows is a description of some of the more common signs indicating the presence of gallstones in the liver and gallbladder. If you have any of them, you will most likely derive great benefits from cleansing your liver and gallbladder. In my practice, I have found these indications to be highly accurate. In case you are not sure whether you have stones, it may be useful to cleanse the liver anyway; it can improve your health significantly, regardless. There is an old saying: "The proof of the pudding is in the eating." The only way to discover for yourself whether you have gallstones is to do the liver flush. You will find that when you remove all the stones that may be present, the symptoms of disease will gradually disappear, and health will return to normal.

Signs and Marks

The Skin

The major function of the skin is to continuously adjust our internal body to the ever-changing external environment, which includes temperature, humidity, dryness, and light. In addition, skin covers the body to protect us against injury, microbes, and other harmful agents. Apart from having to deal with these *external* influences, the skin also monitors and adapts according to *internal* changes taking place within the body. Accordingly, the skin reflects the condition of the organs and body fluids, including the blood and lymph. Any long-term abnormal functioning of the body will inevitably show up in the skin as skin blemishes, discoloration, or changed condition, such as dryness, oiliness, wrinkles, lines, and so forth. Almost all skin disorders have their root in an imbalanced liver condition. Gallstones lead to circulatory disorders, which reduce the nutrient supply to, and waste removal from, the skin and prevent healthy development and normal turnover cycles of skin cells. The following marks are particularly indicative of gallstones in the liver and gallbladder:

⇒ **Black spots and small or large brown patches** that are the color of freckles or moles. They usually appear on the right or left side of the forehead, between the eyebrows or under the eyes. They may also show up just above the right shoulder or between the shoulder blades. Most prominent are the so-called *liver spots* on the back of the hands and forearms, often seen among middle-aged and elderly people. If gallstones, which are spontaneously excreted by the gallbladder, get caught in the colon, such spots may also appear in the area where the thumb and index finger meet. These liver spots usually start fading after the majority of stones are removed from the liver and gallbladder. Most people assume that the liver spots are due to sun damage and "normal" aging. This is a myth. Liver spots, as the name suggests, come from the liver. Sun exposure merely brings to the surface of the skin any existing acidic waste deposits.

⇒ **Vertical wrinkles between the eyebrows.** There may be one deep line or two, sometimes three, lines in this region. These lines or wrinkles, which are *not* a part of natural aging, indicate an accumulation of many gallstones in the liver. They show that the liver is enlarged and has hardened. The deeper and longer the wrinkles are, the more the deterioration of liver function has progressed. A line

64

near the right eyebrow also indicates congestion in the spleen. Furthermore, the vertical lines represent a great deal of repressed frustration and anger. Anger arises when gallstones prevent proper bile flow. A bilious nature is one that keeps toxins trapped—toxins that the liver tries to eliminate via bile. Vice versa, anger can trigger gallstone formation. If white or yellow patches accompany the wrinkles, a cyst or tumor may be developing in the liver. **Pimples or growth of hair between eyebrows**, with or without wrinkles, indicate that the liver, gallbladder, and spleen are affected.

⇒ **Horizontal wrinkles across the bridge of the nose.** These are a sign of pancreatic disorders due to gallstones in the liver. If a line is deep and pronounced, there may be pancreatitis or diabetes.

⇒ **Green or dark color of the temple area at the sides of the head.** This shows that the liver, gallbladder, pancreas, and spleen are underactive because of deposits of gallstones in both the liver and gallbladder. This may be accompanied by a **green or blue color** on either side of the bridge of the nose, which indicates impaired spleen functions. A **horizontal line** across the bridge of the nose implies weakness of the pancreas.

⇒ **Oily skin in the area of the forehead.** This reflects poor liver performance due to gallstones. The same applies to **excessive perspiration** in this part of the head. A **yellow color of the facial skin** indicates disorders of the bile functions of the liver and gallbladder, and a weakness of the pancreas, kidneys, and excretory organs.

⇒ **Hair loss in the central region of the head.** This mark indicates that the liver, heart, small intestines, pancreas, and reproductive organs are becoming increasingly congested and aggravated. There is a tendency to develop cardiovascular disease, chronic digestive problems, and the formation of cysts and tumors. Early graying of hair shows that liver and gallbladder functions are underactive.

The Nose

⇒ **Hardening and thickening at the tip of the nose.** This indicates chronic liver weakness, resulting in hardening of the arteries and the accumulation of fat around the heart, liver, spleen, kidneys, and prostate glands. If the enlargement is excessive and blood vessels are visible, a heart attack or stroke may be imminent.

⇒ **The nose is constantly red.** This condition shows an abnormal condition of the heart, with a tendency toward high blood pressure (hypertension). A purple nose indicates low blood pressure. Both conditions are due to imbalanced liver, digestive, and kidney functions.

⇒ **Cleft nose or indentation of the tip of the nose.** This mark indicates irregular heartbeat and heart murmur. If one half of the cleft nose is larger than the other, this shows that one side of the heart is abnormally enlarged. **Arrhythmia** and **panic attacks** may accompany this condition. There may be severe lymphatic congestion caused by digestive disorders such as constipation, colitis, stomach ulcer, and so on. Liver functions are subdued because of large amounts of gallstones cutting off the blood supply to the liver cells. Bile secretions are insufficient. (*Note:* I have personally seen clefts in the nose disappear after liver flushing.)

⇒ **The nose is bending toward the left.** Unless caused by an accident, this asymmetric shape of the nose implies that the organs on the right side of the body are underactive. These include the liver, gallbladder, right kidney, ascending colon, right ovary or testicle, and right side of the brain. The main cause of this condition is an accumulation of gallstones in the liver and gallbladder (the nose is likely to return to center once the stones are removed).

The Eyes

⇒ **Skin color under the eyes is yellowish.** This indicates that the liver and gallbladder are overactive. A **dark,** even **black color** in the same area results when the kidneys, bladder, and reproductive organs are overtaxed because of a prolonged disorder of the digestive system. A **grayish, pale color** occurs if the kidneys and, occasionally, the lungs are malfunctioning owing to improper lymph drainage from these organs. Also, the endocrine system may be affected.

⇒ **Water-containing bags under the lower eyelids.** These are formed as a result of congestion in the digestive and excretory organs, which results in inadequate lymph drainage from the head area. If these eye bags are chronic and contain fat, this points toward the presence of inflammation, cysts and, possibly, tumors in the bladder, ovaries, fallopian tubes, uterus, and prostate.

⇒ **A white cloud covers the pupil of the eye.** The cloud consists mostly of mucus and degenerate protein particles. It indicates the development of cataracts brought about by longstanding poor liver and digestive performance.

⇒ **Constant redness in the white of the eye.** This condition is caused by the protrusion of capillaries, indicating disorders in the circulatory and respiratory functions. **White or yellow mucus patches** in the white of the eye show that the body is accumulating abnormal amounts of fatty substances because the liver and gallbladder have amassed large quantities of gallstones. When this occurs, the body has a tendency to develop cysts and both benign and malignant tumors.

⇒ **A thick white line covers parts of the periphery of the**

iris, particularly the lower parts. This indicates the accumulation of large amounts of cholesterol in the blood circulatory system. The lymphatic system also has major congestion and fat retention. (*Note:* If you wish to understand the connection of the eyes and iris with the various parts of the body, I recommend that you study the science of *iridology,* or eye interpretation.)

⇒ **The eyes have lost their natural luster and shininess.** This signals that both the liver and kidneys are congested and unable to filter the blood properly. "Dirty" blood, loaded with toxins or waste products, is heavier and more sluggish than clean blood. The thickened blood slows circulation and reduces oxygen and nutrient supply to the cells and organs, including the eyes. If this condition persists, the cells will deteriorate and inevitably age or die off. The eye and brain cells are especially affected because the blood has to flow against gravity to reach them. **Most vision problems** are the direct or indirect result of reduced blood-cleansing capacity by the liver and kidneys. Clean and nutrient-rich blood from a healthy, efficient liver can flow easily and nourish the eye tissues better, thereby improving most eye problems.

The Tongue, Mouth, Lips, and Teeth

⇒ **The tongue is coated yellow or white, especially in the back part.** This indicates an imbalance in the secretion of bile, which is the major cause of digestive trouble. Toxic residues of undigested and fermented or putrefied food linger in the intestinal tract. This blocks lymph flow in the thoracic duct and prevents toxins and microbes in the throat and mouth area from being removed.

⇒ **Teeth impressions on the sides of the tongue, often accompanied by white mucus discharge.** This indicates weak digestion and inadequate absorption of nutrients from the small intestine.

⇒ **Pimples on the tongue.** They are indicative of poor digestion and the presence of fermenting and putrefying food in both the small and large intestines.

⇒ **Cracks on the tongue.** These are signs of long-term intestinal trouble. When food is not being mixed with a sufficient amount of bile, it remains partially undigested. Undigested foods are subjected to bacterial putrefaction and, thereby, become a source of toxicity. Constant exposure of the intestinal wall to the toxins that these bacteria produce irritates and injures it. The resulting lesions, scars, and hardening of the intestinal walls is then reflected by the cracks on the tongue. There may be little or no mucus discharge on the tongue.

⇒ **Repeated mucus discharge into the throat and mouth.** Bile may regurgitate into the stomach, thereby irritating its protective lining and causing excessive mucus production. Some of the bile and mucus may reach the mouth area. This can create a bad (bitter) taste in the mouth and give rise to frequent attempts at clearing the throat, which sometimes involve coughing. Mucus discharge without this bitter taste results when food is not digested properly, and toxins are generated. The mucus helps to trap and neutralize some of these toxins, but as a side effect, it causes congestion.

⇒ **Bad breath and frequent burping.** Both signs point toward the presence of undigested, fermenting, or putrefying food in the GI tract. Bacteria acting on the waste material produce gases, which can be very toxic at times, hence the bad odor emanating from the breath.

⇒ **Crust formations at the corners of the mouth.** This indicates the presence of duodenal ulcers, caused by regurgitation of bile into the stomach, or by other reasons discussed earlier. **Ulcers** in various parts of the mouth or on the tongue show that inflammation or ulceration is occurring in the corresponding parts of the GI tract. For example, a mouth ulcer on the outside parts of your lower lip points to the presence of ulcer lesions in the large intestine. Herpes ("cold sores") on the lip corresponds to more severe inflammation and ulceration of the intestinal wall.

⇒ **Dark spots or patches on the lips.** These marks occur when obstructions in the liver, gallbladder, and kidneys have resulted in slowness and stagnation of blood circulation and lymph drainage throughout the body. There may be advanced, abnormal constriction of blood capillaries. If the color of the lips is reddish (dark) or purple, this indicates that heart, lung, and respiratory functions are subdued.

⇒ **Swollen or expanded lips.** This condition indicates intestinal disorders. If the lower lip is swollen, the colon suffers constipation, diarrhea, or both, alternating between them. Toxic gases are formed from improperly digested foods, which gives rise to bloating and abdominal discomfort. A swollen or enlarged upper lip indicates stomach problems, including indigestion, frequently accompanied by "heartburn." An abnormal, tightly closed mouth shows that a person suffers from disorders of the liver, gallbladder, and, possibly, the kidneys. If the lower lip is dry, peels, and splits easily, there may either be chronic constipation or diarrhea, with large amounts of toxic acids prevalent in the colon. This condition is accompanied by advanced dehydration of the colon cells.

⇒ **Swollen, sensitive, or bleeding gums.** Any these symptoms occurs when lymph drainage from the mouth area is inefficient as a result of intestinal lymph congestion. The blood has an overload of acid compounds. Inflammation deep in the throat, with or without swelling of the tonsils, is also caused by lymphatic blockage. **Tonsillitis,** which often occurs among children, is a sign of constant retention of toxins contained in the lymph fluids and back-flushing of waste from the GI tract into the tonsils.

⇒ **Tooth problems** are generally caused by nutritional imbalance. Poor digestion and overconsumption of refined, processed, and highly acid-forming foods, such as sugar, chocolate, meat, cheese, coffee, soda, and so forth, deplete the body of minerals and vitamins. Adults usually have thirty-two teeth. Each tooth corresponds to a vertebra of the spine, and each vertebra is connected to a major organ or gland. If any of the four canines are decaying, for example, it indicates the presence of gallstones in the liver and gallbladder. A yellow color of the teeth, and of the canines in particular, indicates the presence of toxins in the organs located in the midabdominal region, that is, the liver, gallbladder, stomach, pancreas, and spleen. Bacteria are *not* the cause of tooth decay. They only attack tooth tissue that already has an unbalanced acid-alkaline ratio. Proper saliva secretions also play a major role in the protection of the teeth. Truly healthy teeth last a lifetime and are maintained by a healthy digestive system.

Hands, Nails, and Feet

⇒ **White, fatty skin on the fingertips** is a sign of dysfunctional digestive and lymphatic systems. In addition, the liver and kidneys may be forming cysts and tumors. An excessive discharge of fats may occur, seen as oiliness on the skin.

⇒ **Dark red fingernails** point toward a high content of cholesterol, fatty acids, and minerals in the blood. The liver, gallbladder, and spleen are congested and underactive, and all excretory functions are overburdened with waste products. **Whitish nails** indicate the accumulation of fat and mucus in and around the heart, liver, pancreas, prostate, or ovaries. This condition is accompanied by poor blood circulation and low hemoglobin levels (anemia).

⇒ **Vertical ridges in the fingernails** generally indicate poor absorption of food and the disruption of important digestive, liver, and kidney functions. There may be general fatigue. Strong vertical ridges on the thumbnails, possibly with split ends, show that a person's testicles and prostate or ovaries are not functioning properly. This is caused by the ineffectiveness of the digestive and circulatory systems. **Horizontal indentations in the nails** show unusual or drastic changes in dietary habits. The changes can be either beneficial or harmful. **White dots on the nails** appear when the body eliminates large amounts of calcium and/or zinc in response to excessive consumption of sugar or sugar-containing foods and beverages. Sugar has highly acid-forming properties and leaches out these minerals from the bones and teeth.

⇒ **A hard protrusion at the ball of the foot.** This condition shows progressive hardening of the organs located in the middle of the body, including the liver, stomach, pancreas, and spleen. It points to the accumulation of numerous gallstones in the liver and gallbladder.

⇒ **A yellow color of the feet** indicates the accumulation of many gallstones in the liver and gallbladder. If the color of any part of the feet is green, then spleen and lymph functions are severely disrupted. This may lead to cysts and to benign and malignant tumors.

⇒ **Hardness at the tip of the fourth toe or a callus in the area under the fourth toe.** This symptom shows that gallbladder functions are stagnant. General rigidity, a bent condition, and pain in the fourth toe imply a long history of gallstones in the gallbladder and liver.

⇒ **Curving of the first toe.** If the large toe curves inward toward the second toe, it shows that liver functions are subdued owing to the presence of gallstones in the liver bile ducts. At the same time, spleen and lymphatic functions are overactive because of the accumulation of toxic residues from inadequately digested foods, metabolic waste, and cellular debris.

⇒ **White color and rugged surfaces on the fourth and fifth toenails.** This indicates poor performance of the liver and gallbladder, as well as of the kidneys and urinary bladder.

The Constitution of Fecal Matter

⇒ **The stool or fecal matter emits a sharp, sour, or penetrative odor.** This indicates that food is not being digested properly. Fermented and putrefied food and the presence of large quantities of "unfriendly" bacteria in the feces give rise to an abnormal odor and sticky texture. Normal stool is coated with a thin mucus lining, which prevents the anus from being soiled.

⇒ **Dry and hard stools** are an indication of constipation, and so are sticky stools. Diarrhea is yet another sign of weak performance of the digestive system and the liver, in particular.

⇒ **The feces look pale or clay-colored.** This is still another indication of poor liver performance (bile gives the stool its natural brown color). If the stool floats, large amounts of undigested fats are contained in it, making it lighter than water.

Conclusion

There may be many more signs and symptoms indicating the presence of gallstones in the liver and gallbladder than those listed above. Pain in the right shoulder, tennis elbow, frozen shoulder, numbness in the legs, and sciatica, for example, may have no obvious relation to gallstones in the liver. Yet when the gallstones are removed, these conditions usually disappear.

The body is a network of information, and every part influences and communicates with every other part. Seemingly insignificant marks or signs on the skin, in the eyes, or on a toe may be the harbingers of serious health issues. When you recognize them and flush your liver and gallbladder, in concert with adopting a healthy regimen of diet and lifestyle, you will find that the signs of wellness and vitality begin to reappear. To prevent illness and make permanent health a practical reality in your life, it is important to understand what actually causes gallstones in the first place.

Chapter 3

The Most Common Causes of Gallstones

B ile consists of water, mucus, bile pigment (bilirubin), bile salts, and cholesterol, as well as enzymes and beneficial bacteria. Liver cells secrete this yellow, green, or brownish fluid into tiny canals, known as *bile canaliculi.* The bile canaliculi join up to form larger canals that, in turn, connect with the *right and left hepatic ducts.* The two hepatic ducts combine and form the *common bile duct,* which drains bile from the liver and supplies the gallbladder with the right amount of bile for the process of digestion.

Any abnormal change in the composition of bile affects the solubility of its constituents and, hence, causes gallstones. For simplicity's sake, I have categorized gallstones into two basic types: *cholesterol stones* and *pigment stones.* Some cholesterol stones are composed of at least 60 percent cholesterol and have a yellowish or tan color. Others have a pea-green color and are generally soft, like putty (these can consist of up to 95 percent cholesterol). Some stones may contain other organic, fatty material. *Pigment stones* are brown or black, owing to their high content of colored pigment (bilirubin). They may be calcified, and they are harder and more solid than cholesterol stones. However, cholesterol-based stones can also become hard and calcified. Calcified stones grow only in the gallbladder.

An abnormal alteration of the components of bile can occur in a number of ways. The dissolving action of bile salts and, of course, copious amounts of water, normally keep cholesterol in liquid form. An increased amount of cholesterol in the bile overwhelms the dissolving capacity of the bile salts, thereby promoting the formation of cholesterol stones. Similarly, a decrease in the amount of bile salts being produced also leads to cholesterol stone formation. In addition, due to insufficient water intake, the fluidity of bile decreases, and much of the cholesterol is not dissolved properly; instead it reconstitutes into small cholesterol pebbles. In time, these small pebbles grow into larger ones.

Pigment stones form when the bile pigment, bilirubin, a waste product of the breakdown of red blood cells, increases in the bile. People with excessive amounts of cholesterol stones in the liver are at risk for developing liver cirrhosis, sickle-cell anemia, or other blood diseases. Any of these complications can produce high concentrations of bilirubin pigment in the bile. These abnormally elevated bilirubin levels lead to the formation of pigment stones in the liver and gallbladder.

When the composition of bile in the liver is no longer balanced, small cholesterol crystals begin to combine with other bile components to form tiny clots. These tiny clots can obstruct the even tinier bile canaliculi. This slows the bile flow further, causing more and more bile to attach itself to these tiny clots. Eventually, the clots become large enough to be called stones. Some of these stones may pass into the larger bile ducts and cluster together with other stones. They may also grow to larger-sized stones themselves. The result is that bile flow becomes increasingly obstructed in the larger bile ducts as well. Once several of the larger bile ducts are congested, hundreds of smaller ducts are similarly affected, which closes the vicious cycle. Eventually, the hepatic ducts are so severely clogged with intrahepatic stones (those that occur inside the liver) that the amount of bile available for the digestive process is drastically reduced. Since the liver continues to produce bile, more and more of it is being converted into stones while some of it ends up in the blood. Once bile has leaked into the blood, it may lead to a discoloration of the skin (yellow or gray) and cause skin blemishes, such as liver spots.

Sluggish bile flow in the liver alters the composition of bile still further, which, in turn, affects the gallbladder. A small clot of bile in the gallbladder may take as long as eight years to grow large enough to be noticeable and become a serious health threat. It is known that one in ten Americans has gallstones in the gallbladder. Of these, 500,000 opt for gallbladder surgery each year. Very few physicians and patients, however, are aware of the fact that almost every person with any kind of persistent health problem has gallstones in the liver. It is estimated that about 95 percent of adults in industrialized nations have gallstones in the biliary system of their liver.

Gallstones in the liver can cause many more diseases than gallstones in the gallbladder. To prevent illness and to generate a genuine and lasting breakthrough in the understanding and treatment of disease, we need to have a clear understanding of what dehydrates the bile fluid, alters its natural flora, destroys its enzymes, and increases its cholesterol and bilirubin content. The following four categories shed light on the most common factors responsible for causing gallstones.

Dietary

Overeating

Dietary mistakes probably play the biggest role in producing imbalanced bile composition and, consequently, gallstones. Among all dietary blunders, *overeating* affects health most severely. By regularly eating too much food or eating food more frequently than the body needs to nourish and sustain itself, the digestive juices (including bile) become increasingly depleted. This leaves large proportions of the ingested foods improperly digested. Undigested food putrefies and ferments, becoming a constant source of harmful microbial activity. This rather unnatural means of breaking down food alters the pH (acid-alkaline balance) of the intestinal environment, turning it into a favorable environment for yeast growth and parasites. (*Note:* Cleansing of the liver and colon, and eating a balanced diet rich in fresh, alkaline-forming foods, are among the most effective approaches to prevent and treat parasitic infestation; the killing of parasites does not address its cause and may only have limited benefits, if any.) As more and more toxic substances begin to accumulate or linger in the intestinal tract, the lymph and blood start absorbing some of these harmful substances. This leads to progressive congestion of the lymphatic system and thickening of the blood. All of this overtaxes the liver and excretory functions.

Intestinal disorders can greatly deplete bile salts in the body owing to poor reabsorption from the lower parts of the small intestine. Low levels of bile salt lead to the formation of gallstones. This is clearly shown by the markedly increased risk of gallstones among patients suffering from *Crohn's disease* and other forms of *irritable bowel syndrome.*

An imbalanced blood and lymph condition, caused by overeating, leads to decreased blood flow in the liver lobules, thereby altering bile composition and producing gallstones. Gallstones in the liver further congest the blood and lymph, which upsets the body's basic metabolism. The more one overeats, the fewer nutrients become available to the cells of the body. In fact, constant overeating leads to cell starvation, which creates the strong urge to eat food more often than is normal. The repeated desire to snack, known as food craving, is a sign of serious malnourishment and metabolic imbalance. Moreover, it indicates imbalanced liver activity and the presence of gallstones.

Eating to the point at which you feel completely full, or feel that you cannot eat any more food, is a clear signal that the stomach has reached the point of dysfunction. Digestive juices in the stomach are only able to combine with ingested food as long as the stomach is at least one-quarter empty. Two cupped handfuls of food (use your own hands to measure) equal about three-quarters the size of your stomach. This is the maximum amount of food the stomach can process at one time. Therefore, it is best to stop eating when you reach the point at which you feel you could still eat a little more. Leaving the dinner table slightly hungry greatly improves digestive functions and prevents gallstones and disease from arising.

Eating Between Meals

Ayurveda, the most ancient of all health sciences, considers *"eating before the previous meal has been digested"* to be one of the major causes of illness. The following factors are among the more common reasons why people eat in between meals:

⇒ A stressful and hurried lifestyle.

⇒ The temptation generated by the huge variety of processed, refined, and attractively packaged foodstuffs available.

⇒ The convenience of having fast food meals (low in nutritional value) available at virtually any time of the day or night.

⇒ Lack of satisfaction and nourishment from foods eaten; hence, food cravings develop. This can be expressed by the urge to eat popcorn or junk food while watching a movie.

⇒ Emotional eating to comfort oneself and avoid dealing with fear or insecurity issues.

Any or all of these may have contributed to the irregular eating habits prevalent in a large percentage of today's population. As a rule, the more processed and altered foods are, the fewer nutrients and less life energy (Chi) they contain. Since the nutritional value of such foods is so low, we need to eat more in order to satisfy the daily requirements of the body. (*Note:* Taking food supplements can neither replace real food nor provide the satisfaction that arises from eating, which is what the body requires to successfully digest and process nutrients.)

Irregular eating habits, which include eating between meals and snacking in the middle of the night, greatly upset the body's finely tuned biological rhythms.[13] Most of the important hormonal secretions in the body depend on regular cycles of eating, sleeping, and waking. For example, the production of bile and intestinal digestive juices, which are necessary for breaking down foods into their basic nutrient components, naturally peaks during midday. This suggests that the biggest meal is best eaten around that time. In contrast, the body's digestive capacity is considerably lower during the morning and evening hours. If, day after day, the lunch meal consists merely of light snacks, the gallbladder cannot squeeze *all* its contents into the intestines, so it leaves behind enough bile to form gallstones. Note that the gallbladder is naturally programmed to release the maximum amount of bile during the midday period. If you don't use what the body produces naturally, it can turn on itself.

---

[13] See more details about biological rhythms in the author's book, *Timeless Secrets of Health and Rejuvenation.*

In addition, eating only nonsubstantial meals during lunchtime causes nutritional deficiencies that most often manifest themselves as a frequent urge for foods or beverages that promise a quick energy boost. These include sweets, pastries, breads and pastas made from white flour (starches act like white sugar), chocolate, coffee, black tea, soda, and the like. For every little snack eaten, the gallbladder releases a small amount of bile. However, the secretion of just a little bile is not sufficient to completely empty the gallbladder, which raises the risk of gallstone formation.

Having a constant urge to eat between meals suggests a major imbalance of the digestive and metabolic functions. If you decide to eat something an hour or two after a meal, for example, the stomach is forced to leave the previously eaten meal half-digested and attend to the newly ingested food instead. The older food begins to ferment and putrefy, thereby becoming a source of toxins in the digestive tract. The new food, by contrast, receives inadequate amounts of digestive juices, leaving it only half-digested as well. While the body is engaged in digesting a meal, it is simply incapable of producing and delivering sufficient amounts of bile and other digestive juices to properly handle another meal at the same time. If this stop-and-go process is repeated many times, it results in the generation of ever-increasing amounts of toxins, even as ever-decreasing amounts of nutrients reach the body's cells. Both these stressful situations cause a reduction in bile salts (poor digestion of food decreases the reabsorption of bile salts) and an increase of cholesterol production by the liver in response to poor digestion of fats. Both these situations leave the body with no other choice but to produce gallstones.

To escape this vicious cycle, allow yourself to go through the initial phases of food cravings with more awareness. Feel what your body is "telling you" when it signals discomfort. Ask yourself what your body *really* wants. If you crave something sweet, try eating a piece of fruit instead.

In many people, the urge to eat is actually a sign of dehydration, and all the body really wants is water. Because hunger and thirst signals are identical, the hunger pang or discomfort may subside once you drink one or two glasses of water. At the same time, make certain that you get a substantial and nutritious meal at lunchtime. In time, and provided you have completely cleansed your liver, your body will receive enough nutrients from this main meal to satisfy almost all its daily nutritional requirements. This will effectively stop food cravings and the desire to eat in between meals.

Eating Heavy Meals in the Evening

A similar eating disorder occurs when the main meal of the day is consumed in the evening. Secretions of bile and digestive enzymes are drastically reduced later in the afternoon, especially after 6 p.m. For that reason, a meal consisting of foods such as meat, chicken, fish, cheese, or eggs cannot be properly digested later in the day. Oily foods or those fried in oil are too difficult for the body to digest in the evening. Instead, such a meal turns into toxic waste matter in the intestines.

Undigested foods always end up congesting the body, first in the intestinal tract, and then in the lymph and blood. This greatly affects the quality of digestion during daytime meals. Gradually, the digestive power, which is determined by balanced secretions of hydrochloric acid, bile, and digestive enzymes, becomes subdued, causing similar side effects to those that result from overeating. Therefore, eating a large meal in the evening is a major contributing factor in the development of gallstones in the liver. Eating food before going to sleep also upsets the digestive functions, for similar reasons. Ideally, there should be at least three hours between eating and bedtime. The ideal time for evening meals is around 6 p.m., and the ideal bedtime is before 10 p.m.

Overeating Proteins

As mentioned earlier, excessive protein consumption leads to the thickening and congestion of the basal membranes of the blood vessels (capillaries and arteries), including the liver sinusoids.[14]

---

[14] The author's book *Timeless Secrets of Health and Rejuvenation* explains in great detail how overconsumption of protein foods (of any origin) affects the circulatory system, and how reducing proteins in our diet clears the arterial plaque obstructing blood flow to the heart.

Protein deposits in the blood sinusoids hinder serum cholesterol from leaving the bloodstream. Therefore, the liver cells "assume" that there must be a shortage of cholesterol in the body. This perceived "shortage" stimulates the liver cells to raise cholesterol production to abnormally high levels (some of the cholesterol is needed to heal and protect injured parts of the arteries). This extra cholesterol enters the liver bile ducts with the intention of being taken to the small intestines for absorption. However, because the membranes and openings of the sinusoids are clogged with accumulated protein fiber (collagen), most of the extra cholesterol never makes it there and, instead, is caught in the bile ducts. Any excessive cholesterol (not combined with bile salts) forms small clumps of crystals that combine with other bile components in the liver and gallbladder. This is how cholesterol stones are made.

Interestingly, Asians generally have a low-protein but high-fat diet, and rarely have cholesterol stones in their gallbladders. On the other hand, cholesterol stones in the gallbladder are very common among Americans whose diet is rich in flesh and milk protein.

Dietary fats play only a secondary, almost insignificant, role in raising cholesterol levels in the blood. The liver cells produce most of the cholesterol the body requires on a daily basis for the normal metabolic processes. The main reason we need fats in our diet is not so much to meet our need for cholesterol, but to help digest and absorb other foods and to derive fat-soluble vitamins. The liver raises cholesterol production to abnormal levels only when the basal membranes of the sinusoids are plastered with protein deposits.

Other factors that generate excessive amounts of protein in the blood include stress, smoking, and drinking alcohol and caffeinated beverages. Smoking, for example, causes inhaled carbon monoxide to destroy red blood cells, thus unleashing a large amount of protein particles into the blood. Once enough of these degenerate proteins are deposited in the blood vessel walls, adequate quantities of cholesterol can no longer reach the body's cells, and the liver cells automatically raise cholesterol production. The side effect of this response is gallstone formation.

If you are not a vegetarian, it is best to cut out meat,[15] eggs, and cheese first, and keep other types of animal protein, such poultry and fish, to a minimum. Although all animal-based protein has a gallstone-generating effect, white meat, including chicken, turkey, and rabbit, causes a little less damage to the liver, provided they are of free-range origin and not eaten more often than once or twice a week.[16] It is best to avoid fried and deep-fried foods, as they aggravate both the gallbladder and the liver. Once your taste for meat or other animal proteins begins to diminish, you can gradually switch to a balanced vegan diet.

Over two-thirds of the world's population are still vegetarian (they eat some dairy) or vegan (they eat nothing from animals) and, therefore, they consume little or no animal protein. These population groups show almost no signs of such degenerative illnesses as heart disease, cancer, osteoporosis, arthritis, diabetes, obesity, MS, and the like.

The body's protein requirements are actually quite small, and certainly not as high as you have been led to believe by the food and medical industries. First, about 95 percent of the body's protein is recycled. Second, the liver synthesizes new proteins from amino acids that are not necessarily derived from the foods you eat. In fact, each cell in the body makes proteins. The nucleus of each cell is constantly engaged in protein production. Brain cells produce proteins, known as *neuropeptides*, in response to every thought or feeling you have. Neuropeptides, also known as *neurotransmitters,* are the molecular language that allows mind, body, and emotions to communicate. The body makes thousands of different enzymes, all of which consist of proteins. Not eating

---

[15] According to the latest results (Nov. 2006) of The Nurses' Health Study, which is among the largest prospective investigations into the risk factors for major chronic diseases in women, women double their risk of hormone-receptor-positive breast cancer by eating more more than 1 1/2 servings a day of beef, lamb or pork. A serving is roughly equivalent to a single hamburger or hot dog. If such a small amount of meat can cause cancer, it can surely cause a lot of other health problems as well, including gallstones.

[16] Note that poultry contains the highest concentration of parasites and parasite eggs among animal products. For example, more than 80 percent of all poultry in the United States is infested with salmonella. Cadavers like meat, poultry, and fish are naturally subject to parasitic infestation.

protein foods does not diminish the body's ability to make proteins. On the contrary, overeating proteins can severely congest the blood and lymph and can suffocate cells, thereby diminishing their ability to manufacture proteins. In fact, most protein deficiencies result from eating too much protein.

All proteins are made of various chains of amino acids, and amino acids consist of nitrogen, carbon, hydrogen, and oxygen molecules. These molecules are ingested by the body during inhalation of air. The air is saturated with these four molecules. When you inhale air, you are using not only the oxygen molecules but all the other molecules as well. Since all of these enter the blood right away, they are readily available to all cells in the body. This is the only truly efficient way for the brain cells and all the other cells in the body to be self-sufficient with respect to their protein requirements.

It would be far too complicated, inefficient, and laborious for the body to convert degenerated cadaver-proteins from killed animals into fresh, vital proteins. Heating fish, eggs, meat, and poultry almost completely destroys (coagulates) these proteins, making it very difficult for human cells to use them. If the body depended on eating protein foods on a regular basis, most people in the world would be deathly ill or dead by now. However, this has not happened. On the contrary, the sickest people on the planet live in the United States and other industrialized nations where protein is considered a necessary food. The common assumption that you need to eat protein-rich food daily is not only misleading but also highly unscientific.[17] People on a balanced vegan diet rarely suffer from a chronic illness. A recent study showed that a vegan diet may even reverse diabetes. In addition, it is a myth that vegans are more prone to anemia owing to a deficiency in vitamin B12 than meat-eaters. In fact, I see far more anemic meat-eaters than vegetarians who are anemic. I personally suffered years of childhood anemia while on animal proteins, but completely recovered from it after eight weeks on a vegan diet (with the exception of butter). The idea of having to combine certain foods in order to get complete proteins is plain misinformation, too. The

---

[17] The author has not eaten any concentrated protein food in any form for over thirty-five years and has never suffered from protein deficiency.

body does not depend on food proteins to produce the proteins it requires to be healthy.

The strongest animals like the elephant, wild horse, gorilla, and bull do not have to eat animal proteins either. Like us, their large lungs provide them with the right amounts of molecules to make their own proteins and strong muscles. By giving them animal protein-based feeds, they become sick or die. In addition, consider how plants such as avocados, beans, nuts, and seeds make their proteins. These plants take the nitrogen, hydrogen, carbon, and oxygen molecules (carbon dioxide) from the air. With the help of the sun and water (combined hydrogen and oxygen molecules) and a few minerals from the soil, they make "solid" carbohydrates and proteins. Is our body any less capable of doing the same?

Human breast milk is a newborn child's most important and balanced food. However, in comparison with cow's milk, it contains almost no protein, that is, just about 1.5 percent. Compared with human milk, cow's milk contains three times the amount of protein. Right from the beginning of life, the growing baby is naturally prevented from ingesting a concentrated protein food. There is no need for such a food anyway, since the infant's first breath delivers most of the raw ingredients to jump-start protein synthesis by the cells. It should be noted here that life-long vegans have the lowest incidence of gallstones, heart disease, and cancer.[18]

Other Foods and Beverages

Eggs, pork, greasy food, onions, fowl, pasteurized milk, ice cream, coffee, chocolate, citrus fruits, corn, beans, and nuts—in that order—are known to bring on gallbladder attacks in patients suffering from gallbladder disease. In a 1968 research study, an entire group of patients with gallbladder disease was free of symptoms while on a diet that excluded all these foods. Adding eggs to their diet brought on gallbladder attacks in 93 percent of the patients. Egg protein, in particular, can have a gallstone-

---

[18] To learn more about vegetarianism and a wholesome vegetarian diet according to body type (Ayurvedic), refer to *Timeless Secrets of Health and Rejuvenation.*

producing effect. Researchers believe that the ingestion of substances that cause allergies makes the bile ducts swell up, which, in turn, impedes the discharge of bile from the gallbladder.

This assumption, however, is only partially true. From the Ayurvedic point of view, gallstone formation is a *Pitta disorder*, affecting mostly the Pitta body type, although any body type can suffer a Pitta disorder and produce gallstones. In the ancient language of *Sanskrit*, Pitta literally means *bile*. People of this body type naturally secrete bile in large amounts. However, bile secretions become erratic, excessive, or irregular when the Pitta type eats the above foods in large amounts or on a regular basis. Bile's constituent parts become imbalanced, which predisposes it to hardening. This does not mean, though, that Pitta types are naturally prone to gallbladder disease; rather, it means that the digestive system of these individuals is not designed to digest specific foods that are not conducive for their body's growth and sustenance.

The Pitta body type is known to have only limited amounts of enzymes to break down certain foods and beverages, of which the most prominent are:

Sour dairy products, including cheese, yogurt, and sour cream; egg yolks; salty butter; all nuts except a small amount of almonds, pecans, and walnuts; hot spices, as well as ketchup, mustard, pickles, and refined or processed salt; salad dressings that contain vinegar; spicy condiments (sauces); citrus fruit and juices; all sour and unripe fruits; brown sugar; whole (nonground) grains, such as those contained in many whole wheat breads; brown rice; lentils; alcohol; tobacco; coffee and regular tea; colas and other soft drinks; artificial sweeteners, preservatives, and colorings; most pharmaceutical drugs and narcotics; chocolate and cocoa; leftover, frozen, and microwaved foods; and all iced beverages.

Although the Pitta type is the most prone to develop gallstones, other body types are also at risk if they regularly eat foods that clash with their natural constitutional requirements.[19] In addition, manufactured and preserved foods and beverages disturb liver functions in any body type. Foods that contain artificial

---

[19] For further details about diets according to body types, also refer to *Timeless Secrets of Health and Rejuvenation.*

sweeteners, such as aspartame, Splenda, or saccharine, severely upset the liver, gallbladder, and pancreas. Drinking alcohol on a regular basis has a dehydrating effect on both the bile and the blood, causing fat deposits in the liver; eating foods that contain a lot of sugar has the same effect. Moreover, carbonated drinks and fruit juices are loaded with sugar. The increased consumption of sugar among children may explain why such a high percentage of younger people today already have so many gallstones in the liver, although relatively few children normally develop stones in the gallbladder at such an early age. (I personally know of numerous ill children, who have done liver flushes and released hundreds of gallstones.) Children between the ages of 10 and 16 can do liver flushes at half the adult dosage (apple juice, Epsom salts, olive oil, and juices). Unless they have a small frame, children who are 16 or older can follow the normal directions for adults.

Children rarely produce gallstones if they eat a balanced, vegetarian diet that is rich in vegetables, fruits, and complex carbohydrates.

Effects of Refined and Unrefined Salt

Natural sea salt contains ninety-two essential minerals, whereas refined adulterated salt (a byproduct of the chemical industry) contains only two elements, sodium (Na) and chlorine (Cl). When cells suffer from a dietary deficiency of trace elements, they lose their ability to control their ions. This has dire consequences on the human body. Even if ion equilibrium is lost for just one minute, cells in the body begin to burst. This can lead to nervous disorders, brain damage, or muscle spasms, as well as a breakdown of the cell-regenerating process.

When ingested, natural sea salt (reconstituted seawater) allows liquids to freely cross body membranes, blood vessels walls, and glomeruli (filter units) of the kidneys. Whenever the natural salt concentration rises in the blood, the salt will readily combine with the fluids in the neighboring tissues. This, in turn, will allow the cells to derive more nourishment from the enriched intracellular fluid. In addition, healthy kidneys are able to remove these natural saline fluids, without a problem, which is essential for keeping the fluid concentration in the body balanced. Refined salt, however, may pose a great risk to the body. It prevents this free crossing of liquids and minerals (see the reasons for this below), thereby causing fluids to accumulate and stagnate in the joints, lymphatic ducts and lymph nodes, and kidneys. The dehydrating effect of commercial salt can lead to gallstone formation, weight increase, high blood pressure, and other health problems.

The body requires salt to properly digest carbohydrates. In the presence of natural salt, saliva and gastric secretions are able to break down the fibrous parts of carbohydrate foods. In its dissolved and ionized form, salt facilitates the digestive process and sanitizes the GI tract.

Commercially produced table salt has just the opposite effect. To make salt resist the reabsorption of moisture and, thereby, be more convenient for the consumer, salt manufacturers add chemicals such as desiccants, as well as different bleaches, to the final salt formula. After undergoing processing, the salt can no longer blend or combine with human body fluids. This invariably undermines the most basic chemical and metabolic processes in the body. Water retention and kidney and blood pressure problems are the most obvious consequences of refined salt consumption. Refined salt is still added to thousands of different manufactured foods. Some 50 percent of the American population suffers from water retention (the leading cause of weight gain and obesity). The consumption of large amounts of refined salt is much to blame for that.

Before salt was commercially produced, versus harvested naturally, it was considered the most precious commodity on earth, even more precious than gold. During the Celtic era, salt was used to treat major physical and mental disturbances, severe burns, and other ailments. Research has shown that seawater removes hydroelectrolytic imbalance, a disorder that causes a loss of the immune response, allergies, and numerous other health problems (for more details see *Eat Unrefined Sea Salt* in Chapter 5).

In recent years, salt has earned a bad reputation, and people have learned to fear it, in the same way they fear cholesterol and sunlight. Many doctors warn their patients to stay away from sodium and sodium-rich foods. However, to live a salt-free life means that you will suffer an increased risk of mineral and trace mineral deficiencies, as well as numerous related complications. Eating unrefined salt fulfills the body's need for salt without upsetting the hydroelectrolytic balance. If your diet contains a goodly amount of potassium in natural form, you should have no concern about being harmed by the relatively small amount of sodium in real sea salt. Foods that are particularly high in potassium are bananas, apricots, avocados, pumpkin seeds, beans, potatoes, winter squash, and many other vegetables. However, if potassium levels in the body drop below normal, sodium (even in natural salt) can become a source of imbalance.

Celtic ocean salt (grayish in color) is a particularly good product to ingest because it is naturally extracted through sun drying. Other great salts are sold at whole food stores or co-ops. Some are multicolored; others have a pink color. Himalayan salt is considered the best and most nutritious of all. If taken dissolved in water or added to the water in which foods are cooking, these salts have profound, positive effects at the cellular level. Unrefined salt also helps to cleanse and detoxify the gastrointestinal tract, and it keeps harmful germs at bay.

Dehydration

Many people suffer from dehydration without being aware of it. Dehydration is a condition in which body cells do not receive enough water for basic metabolic processes. The cells may run dry for a number of reasons:

⇒ Lack of water intake (anything less than six glasses of pure water per day)
⇒ Regular consumption of beverages that have diuretic effects, such as coffee, regular tea (black), most soda beverages, and alcohol, including beer and wine. (Herbal teas such as green tea, peppermint tea, and the like, have no diuretic effects; decaffeinated coffee and tea are more harmful than in their caffeinated form.)
⇒ Regular consumption of stimulating foods or substances, such as meat, hot spices, chocolate (except small amounts of dark chocolate), sugar, tobacco, narcotic drugs, soda,

and artificial sweeteners
⇒ Stress
⇒ Most pharmacological drugs
⇒ Excessive exercise
⇒ Overeating and excessive weight gain
⇒ Watching television for several hours each day

Any of these factors has a blood-thickening effect and, thereby, forces cells to give up water. The cell water is used to restore blood thinness. To avoid self-destruction, however, the cells begin to hold on to water. They do this by increasing the thickness of their membranes. Cholesterol, which is a clay-like substance, attaches itself to the cell walls, thereby preventing the loss of cellular water. Although this emergency measure may preserve water and save the cell for the time being, it also reduces the cell's ability to absorb new water, as well as much-needed nutrients. Some of the unabsorbed water and nutrients accumulate in the connective tissues surrounding the cells, causing swelling of the body and water retention in the legs, kidneys, face, eyes, arms, and other parts. This leads to considerable weight gain. At the same time, the blood plasma and lymph fluids become thickened and congested. Dehydration also affects the natural fluidity of bile and, thereby, promotes the formation of gallstones.

Tea, coffee, cola, and chocolate share the same nerve toxin (stimulant), *caffeine*. Caffeine, which is readily released into the blood, triggers a powerful immune response that helps the body to counteract and eliminate this irritant. The toxic irritant stimulates the adrenal glands, and, to some extent, the body's many cells, to release the stress hormones adrenaline and cortisol into the bloodstream. The resultant sudden surge in energy is commonly referred to as "the fight-or-flight response." If consumption of stimulants continues regularly, however, this natural defense response of the body becomes overused and ineffective. The almost constant secretion of stress hormones, which are highly toxic compounds in and of themselves, eventually alters the blood chemistry and causes damage to the immune, endocrine, and nervous systems. Future defense responses are weakened, and the body becomes more prone to infections and other ailments.

The boost in energy experienced after drinking a cup of coffee is not a direct result of the caffeine it contains, but rather of the immune system's attempt get rid of the caffeine. An overexcited and suppressed immune system fails to provide the "energizing" adrenaline and cortisol boosts needed to free the body from the acidic nerve toxin, caffeine. At this stage, people say that they are "used" to a stimulant, such as coffee. So they tend to increase their intake of it to feel the "benefits." The often-heard expression "I am dying for a cup of coffee" reflects the true peril of this situation.

Since the body cells have to sacrifice some of their own water for the removal of the nerve toxin *caffeine,* the regular consumption of coffee, tea, or colas causes them to become dehydrated. For every cup of tea or coffee you drink, the body has to mobilize 2 to 3 cups of water just to remove the stimulants, a luxury it cannot afford. This also applies to soft drinks, medicinal drugs, or any other stimulants, including watching TV for many hours (see more about this in the section on *Miscellaneous Causes* later in this chapter). As a rule, all stimulants have a strong, dehydrating effect on the bile, blood, and digestive juices.

Rapid Weight Loss

Overweight people are at greater risk for developing gallstones than people of average weight. It is an undisputed fact that significant health benefits are gained from losing excess pounds. Many people, for example, can normalize high blood pressure, blood sugar, and cholesterol levels through weight loss.

However, achieving rapid weight loss through diet programs that advise a very low intake of calories each day, increases a person's risk of developing gallstones, in both liver and gallbladder. Some low-calorie diets may not contain enough fat to enable the gallbladder to contract sufficiently to empty its bile. A meal or snack containing approximately 10 grams (one-third of an ounce) of fat is necessary for the gallbladder to contract normally. If this does not happen, the gallbladder retains the bile, which subsequently leads to stone formation.

Obesity is associated with increased cholesterol secretion into the bile ducts, which raises the risk of developing cholesterol stones. When obese individuals undergo rapid or substantial weight loss by following an unbalanced diet program or using diet pills, the congested and, therefore, undernourished body seeks to utilize nutrient and fat components from reserve deposits. This quickly raises blood fats and further increases the risk of gallstone formation. The sudden formation of gallstones among people following rapid weight loss programs appears to be a result of increased cholesterol and decreased bile salts in the bile.

Gallstones are also common among obese patients who lose weight rapidly after gastric bypass surgery. (In gastric bypass surgery, the size of the stomach is reduced, preventing the person from overeating.) One study found that more than one-third (38 percent) of patients who had gastric bypass surgery developed gallstones within three months after the surgery. The research findings, however, refer only to gallstones in the gallbladder. The damage done to the liver itself through this procedure is likely to be far greater than the negative effects that organ suffers as a result of a few gallstones accumulating in the gallbladder.

If substantial or rapid weight loss increases the risk of developing gallstones, the obvious way to reduce this risk is to lose weight more gradually. In fact, this problem is solved when toxic waste deposits, including gallstones, are removed from the body and a balanced lifestyle and appropriate diet are implemented.[20] In such a case, weight loss does not *increase* the risk of gallbladder disease, but *reduces* it. By eliminating all stones from the liver and gallbladder and keeping the intestines clean, an obese person can drastically improve digestive functions and gain a renewed state of vitality. Such an approach cuts out the harmful side effects that may be associated with sudden weight loss.

Low-Fat Diets

The promotion of a low-fat diet as *"the healthiest diet of all"* can be held partly responsible for the continuous increase in liver and gallbladder disease among the populations of the developed

---

[20] For in-depth details, see the author's book Timeless Secrets of Health and Rejuvenation.

nations. Foods high in protein are still heralded as being crucial for the development of physical strength and vitality. Fats, by contrast, have been branded as a culprit for causing many of today's chronic diseases, including atherosclerosis.

At the beginning of the twentieth century, heart attacks were extremely rare anywhere in the world. Since that time, fat consumption, per capita, has remained almost the same. Yet since World War II the consumption of protein has risen most dramatically in the affluent parts of the world. The overconsumption of protein foods in industrialized nations has caused an unprecedented number of circulatory diseases, as well as fatalities resulting from heart attacks. In comparison, these health problems occur only rarely among ethnic groups that consume mostly vegetarian foods. In fact, a report issued by the American Medical Association stated that a vegetarian diet could prevent 97 percent of all cases of thrombosis leading to heart attacks.

Although a balanced vegetarian diet may contain larger amounts of fats, the fats do not seem to have any detrimental effects on the circulatory system (unless, of course, they are contaminated by harmful trans fatty acids). In contrast, overeating proteins of animal origin causes thickening of the liver blood vessels, which leads to gallstone formation in the bile ducts. The presence of gallstones, in turn, reduces bile production in the liver. Diminished bile secretions undermine the body's ability to digest fats. Because of indigestion, possible weight gain, and other discomforts arising from such a condition, doctors tell this type of person to cut down on dietary fats. But this prevents the gallbladder from completely emptying its bile contents, leading to even more problems with fat digestion. Eventually, the body will run short of useful essential fats and fat-soluble vitamins. This prompts the liver to increase cholesterol production, causing yet more gallstones to be formed.

The less fat the body receives with the food, the worse the situation becomes. However, since fats cannot be digested properly anymore, the body enters a vicious cycle, which in most cases can only be stopped by removing *all* gallstones from the liver and gallbladder and then gradually increasing fat intake to normal levels.

Low-fat milk, for example, may be one of the culprits that could start such a vicious cycle. In its natural state, full-fat milk contains the right amount of the fats required to digest milk proteins. Without milk fats, the milk protein remains undigested. When much of the milk fat is removed from the milk, the gallbladder is not stimulated enough to release the right amounts of bile necessary to help digest both the milk proteins and the milk fats. Hence, milk proteins and fats are passed into the GI tract without being digested properly. Much of the protein putrefies, and the fats turn rancid. All this leads to severe lymphatic congestion, as is often seen in the bloated stomachs of formula-fed babies.[21] The babies suffer from intestinal colic. Instead of being lean, their faces are moon-like, and their arms, legs, and stomach are puffy and bloated. These babies are susceptible to colds and other infections, have sleeping problems, and tend to cry a lot. The undigested milk or milk formula may be responsible for the development of gallstones in the livers of very young children. Even the *whole-fat milk* offered in food stores today has a reduced fat content, making milk indigestible for most people.[22]

2. Pharmacological Drugs

Hormone Replacement Therapy and Birth Control Pills

The risk of developing gallstones is four times higher among women than among men. It is especially pronounced among women who have used or use birth control pills and hormone replacement therapy (HRT). According to medical research, oral contraceptives and other *estrogens* double a woman's chance of developing gallstones. The female hormone, *estrogen,* which is

---

[21] Such congestion is also seen in women who are told they need to drink milk to keep their bones strong.

[22] For further details about the dangers involved in eating low-fat or "light" foods, as well as milk, see the author's book Timeless Secrets of Health and Rejuvenation.

contained in contraceptive pills and hormone replacements, increases bile cholesterol and decreases gallbladder contraction. Therefore, this estrogen-effect may be responsible for not only causing gallstones in the liver and gallbladder, but also for many other diseases that arise from diminished liver and gallbladder functions. Earlier medical research also implicated *progestogens* contained in HRT drugs in the development of gallstones.

Women who are going through menopause can find great relief from menopausal symptoms by doing a series of liver flushes. Improved liver performance and an increased production of bile, in particular, can prevent and reverse osteoporosis and other bone/joint problems if diet and lifestyle are also balanced.

Other Pharmaceutical Drugs

Prescription medications used to lower the level of fats (lipids) in the blood, including *clofibrate* (Atromid-S) or similar cholesterol-lowering drugs, actually increase cholesterol concentrations in the bile and, thereby, lead to an increased risk of gallstones. These drugs successfully lower blood fats, which they are designed to do. However, having high blood fats actually implies a shortage of fats. Fats become trapped in the blood when they are unable to cross capillary membranes and are, therefore, lacking in the cells. By lowering blood fats with drugs, the body's cells are starved of fats. This can lead to serious cell degeneration.

Octretide, one of the new generations of "statin" drugs, prevents the gallbladder from emptying itself after a fatty meal, leaving plenty of bile behind to form stones. The dangers involved in such a method of medical intervention are obvious; they are certainly more serious than having raised levels of blood fats. (Contrary to common belief, there is no scientific evidence, to date, that shows high blood fats are responsible for causing heart disease.)

According to several studies published in various medical journals, such as the *Lancet,* certain antibiotics also cause gallstones. One of these is *ceftriaxone,* used to treat lower respiratory tract infections, skin and urinary tract infections, pelvic inflammatory disease, and bone and joint infections, as well as meningitis. Similarly, antirejection drugs given to kidney and heart transplant patients increase the likelihood of gallstone formation. *Thiazides,* which are water pills used to control high blood pressure, may also bring on gallbladder disease in patients with gallstones. Furthermore, children taking *furosemide* (Lasix), used to treat hypertension and edema, are likely to develop gallstones, according to research published in the *Journal of Perinatology. Prostaglandins,* which are also used to treat high blood pressure, have no fewer side effects. Painkillers such as *aspirin* and *tylenol* have recently been shown to raise blood pressure by up to 34 percent and thereby damage the liver and other organs.

All pharmacological drugs are toxic by nature and require detoxification by the liver. Yet, impaired liver function permits many of these poisonous chemicals to enter the bile. This alters the natural balance of its constituents and leads to the development of gallstones in the liver and gallbladder. It is worth mentioning that the above findings refer only to gallstones in the gallbladder and do not reveal the severity of damage that these drugs can cause to the liver itself. If pharmacological drugs are able to generate some gallstones in the gallbladder, we can assume that they produce hundreds, if not thousands, of stones in the liver bile ducts. I repeatedly observed that people who have taken pharmacological drugs in the past have had considerably more gallstones than those who took none.

Symptomatic treatment always has a hefty price tag attached to it, that is, an impairment of basic liver functions. It is far easier and more beneficial for the body to remove all gallstones, restore normal blood values, and improve digestion and waste removal than to suppress the symptoms of a disease. Symptoms are *not* the disease; they only indicate that the body is attempting to save and protect itself. They signal the body's need for attention, support, and care. Treating disease as if it were an enemy, when in reality it is a survival attempt, actually sabotages the body's healing abilities and sows the seeds for further illness.

Fluoride Poisoning

Since the liver is unable to break down fluoride, it attempts to pass this poisonous chemical into the bile ducts (which are the only alternative way for the liver to deal with it). This leads to bile duct congestion and numerous other ailments. Fluoride is added to 60 percent of the drinking water in the United States and a number of other countries. Manufacturers add it to a wide range of products, including soy products, toothpaste, fluoride tablets, fluoride drops, fluoride chewing gum, tea, vaccines, household products, fluoridated salt or milk, anesthetics, mattresses emitting fluoride gases, Teflon, and antibiotics. It is also found in polluted air and polluted ground water. Because of its proven high toxicity, in August 2002 Belgium became the first country in the world to prohibit fluoride supplements.

"Fluoridation … is the greatest fraud that has ever been perpetrated and it has been perpetrated on more people than any other fraud has," said Professor Albert Schatz, Ph.D. (Microbiology), discoverer of *streptomycin* and Nobel Prize winner. Fortunately, 98 percent of Western Europe has rejected water fluoridation. This includes Austria, Belgium, Denmark, Finland, France, Germany, Italy, Luxembourg, the Netherlands, Norway, and Sweden. Exhaustive research has shown that tumors in laboratory animals were found to be the direct result of fluoride ingestion. Other animal studies found that fluoride accumulates in the pineal gland and interferes with its production of melatonin, a hormone that helps regulate the onset of puberty, thyroid functions, and numerous other basic physiological processes. In humans, fluoride has been found to cause arthritis, osteoporosis, hip fractures, cancer, infertility, Alzheimer's disease, and brain damage.

Until the 1950s, European doctors used fluoride to treat hyperthyroidism (overactive thyroid). The daily dose of fluoride that people are now receiving in fluoridated communities far exceeds the dose of fluoride that was found to depress the thyroid gland. Because of fluoridation, millions of people are now suffering from hypothyroidism (underactive thyroid). This condition is currently one of the more common medical problems in the United States. Today, over 150 symptoms can be identified in hypothyroidism. Almost all correlate with known symptoms of fluoride poisoning. The symptoms of hypothyroidism include depression, dizziness, fatigue, weight gain, muscle and joint pain, hair loss, headache, migraine, shortness of breath, GI problems, menstrual problems, unbalanced blood pressure, increased cholesterol levels, allergies, insomnia, panic attacks and moodiness, irregular heart beat, and congestive heart failure. A large number of children and adults in India and other developing countries are crippled and their teeth are destroyed because of fluoride poisoning from industry pollution.

To help the body deal with fluoride-caused illnesses, including hypothyroidism, it is important to clean out the liver bile ducts, avoid fluoride-containing products, and use a water filtering system that removes fluoride. Distillation and reverse osmosis (R/O) are effective in removing the fluoride (along with contaminants). For more ideal filtering devices, you may need to contact your local dealer for water filters or check out my book *Timeless Secrets of Health and Rejuvenation.*

The mineral boron removes fluoride from the body. The most absorbable form of boron is ionic boron, as made available by Eniva, for example (see *Suppliers' List* in Chapter 8). A decongesting diet according to body type[23], regular sleeping and eating habits, and stress-free living conditions are essential for recovery.

3. Lifestyle

Disrupting the Biological Clock

The way we organize and live our lives has a tremendous impact on how the body functions. Its efficiency and performance largely depend on predetermined biological rhythms that are in synchrony with the *circadian rhythms* of nature. Circadian rhythms are closely linked with the movements of our planet around the sun. They are also influenced by the motions of the moon and the other planets in relation to the position of the earth.

Our body follows more than a thousand such 24-hour rhythms. Each individual rhythm controls the timing of an aspect of our

---

[23] See *Timeless Secrets of Health and Rejuvenation* for details on determining your body type and choosing the corresponding foods.

body's functions, including heart rate, blood pressure, body temperature, hormone levels, secretion of digestive juices, and even pain threshold. All these rhythms are well coordinated with one another and are controlled by the brain's "pacemaker device," known as *suprachiasmatic nuclei*. This area of the brain regulates the firing of nerve cells that seem to set the clocks of our biological rhythms. If one rhythm becomes somewhat disrupted, other rhythms are thrown off balance, too. In fact, numerous disorders can arise from interference with one or more of our biological rhythms because of an unbalanced, irregular lifestyle.

This section deals with some of the more common "deviations" that particularly affect the functioning of the liver and gallbladder. By attuning your daily routine to the natural schedule of your body, you can greatly assist it in its ceaseless effort to nourish, cleanse, and heal itself. Moreover, you can also prevent new health problems from arising in the future.

The Natural Sleep/Wake Cycles

The cyclic alternation of night and day regulate our natural sleep/wake cycles as well as various essential biochemical processes. The onset of daylight triggers the release of powerful hormones (*glucocorticoids*), of which the main ones are *cortisol* and *corticosterone*. Their secretion has a marked circadian variation. These hormones regulate some of the more important functions in the body, including metabolism, blood sugar level, and immune responses. Peak levels occur between 4 a.m. and 8 a.m. and gradually decrease as the day continues. The lowest level occurs between midnight and 3 a.m.

By altering your natural daily sleep/wake schedule to a different one, the peak of cortisol's cycle changes as well. For example, if you suddenly start going to sleep after midnight, instead of before 10 p.m., and/or you arise in the morning after 8 or 9 a.m., instead of with or before sunrise at around 6 a.m., you will enforce a hormonal time-shift that can lead to chaotic conditions in the body. Waste materials that tend to accumulate in the rectum and urinary bladder during the night are normally eliminated between 6 and 8 a.m. With a changed sleep/wake cycle, the body has no choice but to hold on to that waste matter and possibly reabsorb a part of it. When you disrupt your natural sleep/wake cycles, the body's biological rhythms desynchronize with the larger circadian rhythms controlled by the regular phases of darkness and light. This can lead to numerous types of disorders, including chronic liver disease, respiratory ailments, and heart trouble.

An upset cortisol cycle can also bring on acute health problems. In the 1980s, researchers discovered that more strokes and heart attacks occur in the morning than at any other time of day. Blood clots form most rapidly at about 8 a.m. Blood pressure also rises in the morning and stays elevated until late afternoon. At around 6 p.m. it drops off, and it hits its lowest level during the night. To support the basic hormonal and circulatory rhythms in the body, it is, therefore, best to go to sleep early (before 10 p.m.) and rise no later than the sun does (ideally at around 6 a.m.). (*Note:* These times change according to the seasons. During the winter, we may need a little more sleep; in the summer, we may need a little less.)

One of the *pineal gland's* most powerful hormones is the neurotransmitter *melatonin*. The secretion of melatonin starts between 9:30 and 10:30 p.m. (depending on age), inducing sleepiness. It reaches peak levels between 1 and 2 a.m. and drops to its lowest levels at midday. The pineal gland controls reproduction, sleep and motor activity, blood pressure, the immune system, the pituitary and thyroid glands, cellular growth, body temperature. and many other vital functions. All of these depend on a balanced melatonin cycle. By going to sleep late or working night shifts, you throw this cycle out of balance, and throw off many other hormonal cycles as well.

Apart from making melatonin, the brain also synthesizes *serotonin,* which is a very important neurotransmitter/hormone related to our state of physical and emotional well-being. It affects day and night rhythms, sexual behavior, memory, appetite, impulsiveness, fear, and even suicidal tendencies. Unlike melatonin, serotonin increases with the light of day; physical exercise and sugar also stimulate it. If you get up late in the morning, the resultant lack of exposure to sufficient amounts of daylight reduces your serotonin levels during the day. Moreover, since melatonin is a breakdown product of serotonin, this habit of rising late also lowers the levels of melatonin during the night.

Any deviation from the circadian rhythms causes abnormal secretions of the important brain hormones melatonin and serotonin. This, in turn, leads to disturbed biological rhythms, which can upset the harmonious functioning of the entire organism, including metabolism and endocrine balance. Suddenly, you may feel "out of synch" and become susceptible to a wide range of disorders, from a simple headache to depression to a fully grown tumor.

The production of growth hormones, which stimulates growth in children and helps maintain muscle and connective tissue in adults, depends on proper sleeping cycles. Sleep triggers growth hormone production. Peak secretion occurs at around 11 p.m., provided you go to sleep before 10 p.m. This short period coincides with dreamless sleep, often referred to as "beauty sleep." It is during this period of the sleep cycle that the body cleanses itself and does its main repair and rejuvenation work. If you are sleep-deprived, growth hormone production drops dramatically. People who work the night shift have a greater incidence of insomnia, infertility, cardiovascular illness, and stomach problems. In addition, performance falls and accident rates are higher during the night.

Natural Mealtimes

Ayurveda, the *Science of Life,* declared thousands of years ago that to maintain physical and emotional well-being, the body must be fed according to a natural time schedule. Like most other functions in the body, the digestive process is controlled by circadian rhythms. The secretions of bile and other digestive juices peak at midday and are at their lowest during the night. For this reason, it is best to eat the largest meal of the day at around midday and take relatively light meals at breakfast and dinner times. This enables the body to digest the ingested food efficiently and absorb the appropriate amount of nutrients necessary for the maintenance of all bodily functions. To avoid interfering with the secretion of digestive juices at lunchtime, it is ideal to eat breakfast no later than 8 a.m. Likewise, to digest your evening meal properly, it is best to eat it no later than 6:30 or 7 p.m.

Any long-term disruption of this cycle, caused either by irregular eating habits or by placing the main emphasis on the evening meal and/or breakfast, leads to the accumulation of undigested foods and congests lymph and blood. This also disturbs the body's natural instincts. If its instincts were intact and functioning properly, we would naturally want to eat only those foods that are suitable for our body type, and we would eat them when we could digest them best. One of the leading causes of gallstone formation is the accumulation of improperly digested foods in the intestinal tract. Eating meals irregularly, or having substantial meals at times of the day when the body is not prepared to produce the appropriate quantities of digestive juices, generates more waste than the body is able to eliminate (also see *Disorders of the Digestive System* in Chapter 1) .

4. Miscellaneous Causes

Watching Television for Several Hours

Scientific research has shown that watching television can dramatically increase cholesterol production in the body. Besides being a necessary component of most tissues and hormones in the body, cholesterol also serves as a stress hormone that increases during physical or mental strain. In fact, cholesterol is one of the first hormones transported to the site of an injury to help heal it. Cholesterol forms an essential constituent of all scar tissue formed during wound healing, whether it is a skin-related injury or a lesion in the wall of an artery.

It can be very tiring and stressful for the brain to compute the fast movement of picture frames for long periods of time. "Television-stress" is especially pronounced among children, whose blood cholesterol can rise by 300 percent within a few hours of watching television. Such excessive secretions of cholesterol alter the composition of bile, which causes the formation of gallstones in the liver.

Exposure to television is a great challenge for the brain. It is far beyond the brain's capacity to process the flood of incoming stimuli that emanate from an overwhelming number of rapidly changing picture frames appearing on the TV screen every split second. The resulting stress and strain takes its toll. Blood pressure rises to help move more oxygen, glucose, cholesterol, vitamins, and other nutrients to various parts of the body, including the brain. All of these are used up rapidly by the heavy brainwork. Add to this the tension associated with the content of some programs—violence, suspense, and the noise of gunshots, cars, and shouting—and the adrenal glands respond with shots of adrenaline to prepare the body for a "fight-or-flight" response. This stress response, in turn, contracts or tightens the large and small blood vessels in the body, causing the cells to suffer a shortage of water, sugar, and other nutrients. This shortage of nutrients, in turn, may create the phenomenon of "insatiable hunger" that so many people experience in front of the television set.

Several kinds of symptoms may result from this effect. You may feel tired, shattered, exhausted, stiff in the neck and shoulders, very thirsty, lethargic, depressed, and even too tired to go to sleep. Stress is known to trigger cholesterol production in the body. Since cholesterol is the basic ingredient of stress hormones, stressful situations use up large quantities of cholesterol to manufacture these hormones. To make up for the loss of cholesterol, the liver raises its production of this precious commodity. If the body did not bother to increase cholesterol levels during such stress encounters, we would have millions of "television deaths" by now. Nevertheless, the stress response comes with a number of side effects, one of which is the formation of gallstones.

Lack of exercise can also lead to stasis in the bile ducts and, thus, cause gallstones.

Emotional Stress

A stressful lifestyle can alter the natural flora (bacteria population) of the bile, thereby causing the formation of gallstones in the liver. One of the leading stress-causing factors in life is not having enough time for oneself. If you do not give yourself sufficient time for the things you must do or want to do, you will feel pressured. Continuous pressure causes frustration, and frustration eventually turns into anger. Anger is an indication of severe stress. It has an extremely taxing effect on the body that can be measured by the amounts of adrenaline and noradrenaline secreted into the blood by the adrenal glands. Under severe stress or excitement, these hormones increase the rate and force of the heartbeat, raise blood pressure, and constrict the blood vessels in the secretory glands of the digestive system. In addition, they restrict the flow of digestive juices, including stomach acids and bile; delay peristaltic movement and the absorption of food; and inhibit the elimination of urine and feces.

When food is no longer digested properly and significant amounts of waste are prevented from leaving the body via the excretory organs, every part of the body becomes affected, including the liver and gallbladder. This congesting effect, resulting from the stress response, gives rise to great discomfort on the cellular level and is felt as emotional upset. Research shows that chronic stress or, rather, the inability to cope with stress, is responsible for 85 to 95 percent of all diseases. These are commonly referred to as *psychosomatic diseases.* Stress-induced obstructions not only require deep physical cleansing, such as liver, colon, and kidney purges, but also require approaches that trigger relaxation.[24]

During relaxation, the body, mind, and emotions move into a mode of performance that supports and enhances all the functions of the body. Contracted blood vessels open again, digestive juices flow, hormones are balanced, and waste is eliminated more easily. Therefore, the best antidote to stress and its harmful effects are methods of relaxation, such as meditation, yoga, spending time in nature, playing with children or pets, playing or listening to music, exercising, walking, and the like. To cope with the fast pace of modern life and to give the nervous system enough time to unwind and release any accumulated tension, it is vital to spend at least 30 to 60 minutes a day by yourself, preferably in silence.

If you have had any stressful periods in your life or currently have difficulties calming down or unwinding, you will greatly benefit from doing a series of liver flushes. Having gallstones in

---

[24] In his book *It's Time to Come Alive,* the author offers profound, effortless methods of relaxation.

the liver is, by itself, a major cause of constant stress in the body. When you eliminate these stones, you will become naturally calm and relaxed. You may also discover that once your liver is clean, you will become much less angry or upset about situations, other people, or yourself, regardless of the circumstances.[25]

Conventional Treatments for Gallstones

Treatments typically used to deal with gallstones aim at either dissolving gallstones directly within the gallbladder or removing the gallbladder through surgery. However, these treatments have no effect whatsoever on the large amount of stones congesting the bile ducts of the liver. It is important to realize that every person who has gallstones in the gallbladder has multiple times as many stones in the liver. The surgical removal of the gallbladder or its stones does *not* substantially increase bile flow, because the stones that are stuck in the liver bile ducts continue to prevent proper bile secretion.

Even in the case of surgical removal of the gallbladder, the situation remains highly problematic for the body. Since the pumping device for bile (the gallbladder) is now gone, the small amount of bile that the liver is able to squirt out through its congested bile ducts comes forth merely in dribbles. Both insufficient bile secretion and the uncontrolled flow of bile into the small intestine continue to cause major problems with the digestion and absorption of food, particularly if it contains fats. The result is an ever-increasing amount of toxic waste that accumulates in the intestinal tract and lymphatic system. The restricted ability to digest and assimilate fats stimulates the liver cells to increase production of cholesterol. The side effect arising from this emergency maneuver of the body is the generation of more gallstones in the liver bile ducts. Therefore, removing the gallbladder is not a solution to digestive problems but, rather, a cause of further and more serious complications in the body, such

---

[25] To fully understand emotions and their root causes and to free yourself from their limitations, refer to the author's book *Lifting the Veil of Duality — Your Guide to Living Without Judgment*.

as cancer and heart disease. Balanced bile secretion, on the other hand, protects the body against most diseases.

Any treatment of the gallbladder, however advanced and sophisticated it may be, can only be considered a drop in the ocean of cure because it does not remove the main problem, which is the hundreds or thousands of gallstones blocking the bile ducts of the liver.

Conventional medicine offers three main approaches to treating gallstones:

⇒ 1. Dissolving Gallstones

For patients with mild, infrequent symptoms, or those who do not want surgery, various drugs are available that claim to dissolve gallstones. On the surface, it seems like a good idea to gradually dissolve gallstones through drugs that contain bile salts (oral dissolution therapy). Given in pill form over a period of twelve months, these drugs may achieve a decrease in cholesterol levels in the bile. But there is no guarantee of this. According to the *British Medical Journal,* the use of bile salts has a failure rate as high as 50 percent. In addition, many "successful" patients simply do not experience complete gallstone dissolution in their gallbladder. For the few patients who do, the recurrence rate can also be as high as 50 percent. Other dissolving agents, such as *methyl tert-butyl ether,* have no advantage over bile salts. Unsuccessful treatment may lead to surgery.

More recently, solvents have been directly instilled into the gallbladder by means of a small catheter placed in the skin. This approach has been shown to be more effective in dissolving cholesterol stones, but it still fails to resolve the major issue—the accumulation of gallstones in the liver. Insufficient scientific research exists to determine what side effects accompany this method of treatment.

⇒ 2. Shock Waves

Another alternative method to surgery is *lithotripsy,* a technique by which the gallstones are literally pounded into submission by a series of sound waves. According to a 1993 report by the medical journal *Lancet,* this therapy has great setbacks because it can result in kidney damage and raise blood pressure – risks that have remained unchanged until today. Both these side effects can lead to an increase in the number of gallstones in the liver (see *Disorders of the Circulatory System* and *Disorders of the Urinary System* in Chapter 1).

In addition, this procedure, in which gallstones are fragmented through shock waves, leaves toxic gallstone residue behind. This residue can quickly become a breeding place for harmful bacteria and parasites and, therefore, infections in the body. Recent studies have confirmed that most patients undergoing this kind of treatment experience internal bleeding, ranging from a small hemorrhage to major blood loss that requires blood transfusion. This treatment also has a high stone-recurrence rate.

⇒ 3. Surgery

In 1996, some 770,000 Americans had their gallbladder removed through surgical intervention. Since then, the number has steadily increased. A gallbladder operation costs between $8,000 and $10,000 and takes about thirty to forth-five minutes with *laproscopy.* While open gallbladder surgery—*cholecystectomy*—is still commonly used for patients with frequent or severe pain, or with a history of acute *cholecystitis,* laparoscopic cholecystectomy has now become the preferred surgical technique. With traditional surgery, the gallbladder is removed through an open technique requiring a standard skin incision and general anesthesia. During laparoscopic cholecystectomy, also called a "keyhole operation," the stone-filled gallbladder is literally pulled through a small incision in the abdomen. Sometimes, open cholecystectomy is required if the keyhole operation fails.

With a keyhole operation, patients seem to recover much faster and often leave the hospital and return to regular activity within days. However, since its introduction, this "Band-Aid" approach to treating gallbladder disease has prompted many patients to have a gallbladder operation unnecessarily; that is, to rid them of some persistent symptoms of discomfort.

Apart from having had no effect on the overall mortality rate from gallbladder diseases, laparoscopic surgery does have its risks. As many as 10 percent of patients coming out of surgery have stones remaining in the bile ducts, according to the *U.S. National Institute of Health.* (*Note:* The bile ducts referred to here are not liver bile ducts). According to *Mayo Health Oasis,* other hazards include lost gallstones in the peritoneal cavity, abdominal adhesion, and possibly infective *endocarditis.* Moreover, according to the *New England Journal of Medicine,* the procedure can cause hemorrhage, inflammation of the pancreas (a potentially fatal condition), and perforation of the duodenal wall. There may also be injury and obstruction of bile ducts and the leakage of bile into the abdomen, increasing the patient's chance of suffering a potentially serious infection. About 1 percent of patients are at risk of dying from this kind of operation.

Bile-duct injuries have increased dramatically because of using keyhole surgery. In Ontario, Canada, where 86 percent of all gallbladder operations are performed in this way, the number of bile duct injuries has risen by over 300 percent since this method has become standard practice in the mid 1990s.

In a number of patients, gallstones are caught in the common bile duct (the main bile duct leading to the duodenum). In such cases, the removal of the gallbladder does not alleviate the symptoms of gallstone disease. To help the condition, a flexible tube is placed in the mouth and advanced to the point where the common bile duct enters the duodenum. During the procedure, the opening of the bile duct is enlarged and the stones are moved into the small intestines. Unfortunately, many of the stones may become stuck in the small or large intestine, becoming a source of constant intestinal infection or related problems.

Conclusion

None of the above procedures addresses the *cause* of gallbladder disease. In fact, they all contribute to further disruption of the digestive and eliminative processes in the body. The short-term relief that a patient may experience after his gallbladder has been removed may mislead the patient to believe that he has been cured. Many others continue to experience the same pain they had when they still had their gallbladder. The continued and often worsened impairment of proper bile secretion by the liver may lead to the development of far more serious health problems than just gallbladder disease.

The following chapter describes a simple procedure that painlessly, safely, and effectively removes not only the few gallstones in the gallbladder, but also, and most importantly, the hundreds and thousands of gallstones in the liver. It is extremely unfortunate that millions of people have had their gallbladder removed unnecessarily or lost their lives because of liver and gallbladder disease. Fortunately, there is a simple, risk-free, inexpensive approach available to every person who wishes to naturally restore liver and gallbladder health and to prevent diseases from arising in the future.

Chapter 4

The Liver and Gallbladder Flush

Cleansing the liver and gallbladder from gallstones is one of the most important and powerful approaches you can take to improve your health. The liver flush requires 6 days of preparation, followed by 16 to 20 hours of actual cleansing. To remove gallstones you need the following items:

Apple juice	Six 32 oz. containers
Epsom salts* (or magnesium citrate)	4 tablespoons dissolved in three 8-oz. glasses of water**
Extra virgin olive oil, cold-pressed	One-half glass (4 oz.)
Either fresh grapefruit (pink is best), or fresh lemon and orange combined***	Enough to squeeze ¾ (6 oz.) glass of juice
2 pint jars, one with a lid	

Note: * Look for Epsom salts (magnesium sulfate). In German-speaking countries it is known as "Bittersalz." For those in the U.S., check out any drugstores or natural food stores. Some packaging labels describe it as a natural laxative. If it is not available, use magnesium citrate.
** I have chosen "glass" instead of "cup" as a measuring unit to avoid confusion about the meaning of "cup" on different continents.
*** If you cannot tolerate grapefruit juice or if it tends to make you nauseated, you may use equal amounts of freshly squeezed lemon and orange juice instead. The effect is the same with either choice.

Preparation

➤ **Drink 1 container of 32 oz. of packaged or freshly prepared apple juice (or see other options below) per day for a period of six days:** (You may drink more than that if it feels comfortable to do so.) The *malic acid* in the apple juice softens the gallstones and makes their passage through the bile ducts smooth and easy. The apple juice has a strong cleansing effect. Some sensitive people may experience bloating and, occasionally, diarrhea during the first few days. Much of the diarrhea is actually stagnant bile, released by the liver and gallbladder (indicated by a brownish, yellow color). The fermenting effect of the juice helps widen the bile ducts. If this becomes somewhat uncomfortable, you can dilute the apple juice with any amount of water, or use other options described later. Drink the apple juice slowly throughout the day, between meals (avoid drinking the juice during, just before, and in the first two hours after meals, and in the evening). This is in addition to your normal water intake of six to eight glasses. *Note:* Preferably, use organic apple juice, although for the purpose of the flush, any good brand of commercial apple juice, apple concentrate, or apple cider works just as well. It may be useful to rinse your mouth out with baking soda and/or brush your teeth several times per day to prevent the acid from damaging your teeth. (In case you are intolerant of apple juice or allergic to it, see the other options explained in *Having Difficulties with the Cleanse* at the end of this chapter.)

➤ **Dietary recommendations:** During the entire week of preparation and cleansing, avoid foods or beverages that are cold or chilled; they chill the liver and, thereby, reduce the effectiveness of the cleanse. All foods or beverages should be warm or at least room temperature. To help the liver prepare for the main part of the cleanse, try to avoid foods from animal sources, dairy products, and fried food items. Otherwise, eat normal meals, but avoid overeating.

➤ **The best times for cleansing:** The main and final part of the liver flush is best done over a weekend, when you are not under any pressure and have enough time to rest. Although the liver flush is effective at any time of the month, it should preferably coincide with a day between full moon and new moon. Try to avoid doing the actual flush on full moon day (the body tends to hold more fluids in the brain and tissues on this day than on others). The day of new moon is the most conducive for cleansing and healing.[26]

➢ **If you take any medication:** While on the liver flush regimen, avoid taking any medication, vitamins, or supplements that are not absolutely necessary. It is important not to give the liver any extra work that could interfere with its cleansing efforts.

➢ **Make sure that you cleanse your colon before and after you do a liver flush:.** Having regular bowel movements is not necessarily an indication that your bowel is unobstructed. Colon cleansing, done either a few days before or, ideally, on the sixth day of preparation, helps to avoid or minimize any discomfort or nausea that may arise during the actual liver flush. It prevents back-flushing of the oil mixture or waste products from the intestinal tract into the stomach. It also assists the body in swiftly eliminating the gallstones. Colonic irrigation (colon hydrotherapy) is the fastest and easiest method to prepare the colon for the liver flush. Colema-board irrigation is the second most preferable method (see details in *Keep Your Colon Clean* in Chapter 5).

➢ **What you need to do on the sixth day of drinking apple juice:** Drink all the 32 ounces of apple juice in the morning. You may start drinking the juice soon after awakening. If you feel hungry in the morning, eat a light breakfast, such as a hot cereal; oatmeal would be an ideal choice. Avoid sugar or other sweeteners, spices, milk, butter, oils, yogurt, cheese, ham, eggs, nuts, pastries, cold cereals, and the like. Fruit or fruit juices are fine. For lunch eat plain cooked or steamed vegetables with white rice (preferably basmati rice) and flavor it with a little unrefined sea or rock salt. To repeat, *do not eat any protein foods, butter, or oil,* or you might feel ill during the actual flush. *Do not eat or drink anything (except water) after 1:30 p.m.,* otherwise you may have difficulties passing

---

[26] For a detailed explanation about lunar influences on the body, see *Timeless Secrets of Health and Rejuvenation.*

stones! Follow the exact schedule below.

The Actual Flush
Evening

6:00 p.m.: Add *4* tablespoons of Epsom salts (magnesium sulfate) to a total of 24 ounces (three 8-oz. glasses) of filtered water in a jar. This makes four 6-oz servings. Drink your first portion (¾ glass) now. You may take a few sips of water afterward to neutralize the bitter taste in your mouth, or may add a little lemon juice to improve the taste. Some people drink it with a large plastic straw to bypass the taste buds on the tongue. Closing the nostrils while drinking it works well for most people. It is also helpful to brush your teeth afterward or rinse out the mouth with baking soda. One of the main actions of Epsom salt is to dilate (widen) the bile ducts, making it easy for the stones to pass. Moreover, the salts clear out waste that may obstruct the release of the stones. (If you are allergic to Epsom salts or are just not able to get them down, you may instead use the second best choice—magnesium citrate—at the same dosage.) Set out the citrus fruit you will be using later, so that it can warm to room temperature.

8:00 p.m.: Drink your second serving (¾ glass) of Epsom salts.

9:30 p.m.: If you have not had a bowel movement until now and have not done a colon cleanse within the past 24 hours, take a water enema; this will trigger a series of bowel movements.[27]

9:45 p.m.: Thoroughly wash the grapefruits (or lemons and oranges). Squeeze them by hand and remove the pulp. You will need ¾ glass of juice. Pour the juice and ½ glass of olive oil into the pint jar. Close the jar tightly and shake hard, about 20 times or until the solution is watery. Ideally, you should drink this mixture

---

[27] For more details on enemas, refer to the author's book *Timeless Secrets of Health and Rejuvenation.*

at 10:00 p.m., but if you feel you still need to visit the bathroom a few more times, you may delay this step for up to 10 minutes.

10:00 p.m.: Stand next to your bed (do not sit down) and drink the concoction, if possible, without interruption. Some people prefer to drink it through a large plastic straw. Drinking it while keeping the nostrils closed seems to work best. If necessary, use a little honey between sips, which helps the mixture go down more smoothly. Most people, though, have no problem drinking in one go. Do not take more than 5 minutes for this (only elderly or weak people may take longer).

PLEASE LIE DOWN IMMEDIATELY!

This is essential for helping to release the gallstones! Turn off the lights and lie flat on your back with one or two pillows propping your head up. Your head should be higher than your abdomen. If this is uncomfortable, lie on your right side with your knees pulled toward your head. **Lie perfectly still for at least 20 minutes, and try not to speak!** Put your attention on your liver. Some people find it beneficial to place a castor oil pack over the liver area.

You may feel the stones traveling along the bile ducts like marbles. There won't be any spasms or pain because the magnesium in the Epsom salts keeps the bile duct valves wide open and relaxed, and the bile that is excreted along with the stones keeps the bile ducts well lubricated. (This is very different than in the case of a gallstone attack where magnesium and bile are not present.) Go to sleep if you can.

If at any time during the night you feel the urge to have a bowel movement, do so. Check if there are already small gallstones (pea-green or tan-colored ones) floating in the toilet. You may feel nauseated during the night and/or in the early morning hours. This is mostly due to a strong, sudden outpouring of gallstones and toxins from the liver and gallbladder, pushing the oil mixture back into the stomach. The nausea will pass as the morning progresses.

The Following Morning

6:00–6:30 a.m.: Upon awakening, but not before 6:00 a.m., drink your third ¾ glass of Epsom salts (if you feel very thirsty, drink a glass of warm water before taking the salts). Rest, read, or meditate. If you are sleepy, you may go back to bed, although it is best if the body stays in an upright position. Most people feel fine and prefer to do some light exercises, such as yoga.

8:00–8:30 a.m.: Drink your fourth and last ¾ glass of Epsom salts.

10:00–10:30 a.m.: You may drink freshly pressed fruit juice at this time. One half-hour later, you may eat one or two pieces of fresh fruit. One hour later you may eat regular (but light) food. By the evening or the next morning you should be back to normal and feel the first signs of improvement. Continue to eat light meals during the following 2-3 days. Remember, your liver and gallbladder have undergone major "surgery," albeit without the harmful side effects or the expense.

Note: Drink water whenever you are thirsty, except right after drinking the Epsom salts and for the first two hours after drinking the oil mixture.

The Results You Can Expect

During the morning and, perhaps, afternoon hours following the liver flush, you will have a number of watery bowel movements. These initially consist of gallstones mixed with food residue, and then just stones mixed with water. Most of the gallstones are pea-green and float in the toilet because they contain bile compounds (see **Figure 13a**). The stones will be in different shades of green and may be bright-colored and shiny like gemstones. Only bile from the liver can cause this green color.

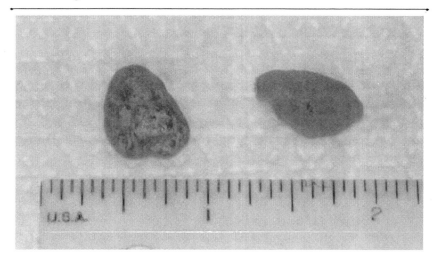

Figure 13a: Green-colored gallstones

Gallstones can come in many sizes, colors, and shapes. The light-colored stones are the newest. Dark-green stones are the oldest. Some are pea-sized or smaller, and others are as big as 1 inch in diameter. There may be dozens and, sometimes, even hundreds of stones (of different sizes and colors) coming out at once (see **Figure 13b**).

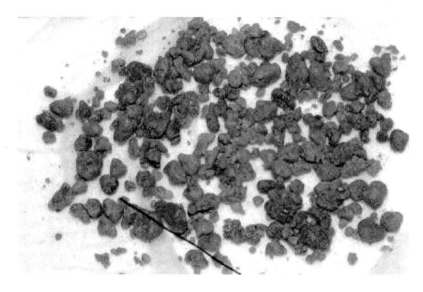

Figure 13b: Mixed types of gallstones

Also, watch for tan-colored and white stones. Some of the larger tan or white stones may sink to the bottom with the stool. These are calcified gallstones that have been released from the gallbladder. They contain heavier toxic substances, with only small amounts of cholesterol (see **Figure 13c**). All the green and yellowish stones are as soft as putty, thanks to the action of the apple juice.

You may also find a layer of white or tan-colored chaff, or "foam," floating in the toilet. The foam consists of millions of tiny white, sharp-edged cholesterol crystals, which can easily rupture small bile ducts. They are equally important to release.

Try to make a rough estimate of how many stones you have eliminated. To permanently cure bursitis, back pain, allergies, or other health problems, and to prevent diseases from arising, you need to remove **all** the stones. This may require at least 8 to 12 flushes, which can be performed at three-week or monthly intervals. *(Do not flush more frequently than that!)* The three-week break between flushes may include the six-day preparation for the next liver flush, but most ideally, it should start after the three weeks have passed. If you cannot flush this often, you may take more time between flushes.

The important thing to remember is that once you have started cleansing the liver, you should keep cleansing it until no more stones come out during two consecutive flushes. Leaving the liver half clean for a long period of time (three or more months) may cause greater discomfort than not cleansing it at all. The liver, as a whole, will begin to function more efficiently soon after the first flush, and you may notice sudden improvements, sometimes within several hours. Pains will lessen, energy will increase, and clarity of mind will improve considerably.

However, within a few days, stones from the rear of the liver will have traveled "forward" toward the two main bile ducts (hepatic ducts) in the liver, which may cause some or all of the previous symptoms of discomfort to return. In fact, you might feel disappointed because the recovery seems so short-lived. Yet all of this merely indicates that some stones were left behind, ready to be removed with the next round of cleansing. Nevertheless, the liver's self-repair and cleansing responses will have increased significantly, adding a great deal of effectiveness to this extremely important organ of the body.

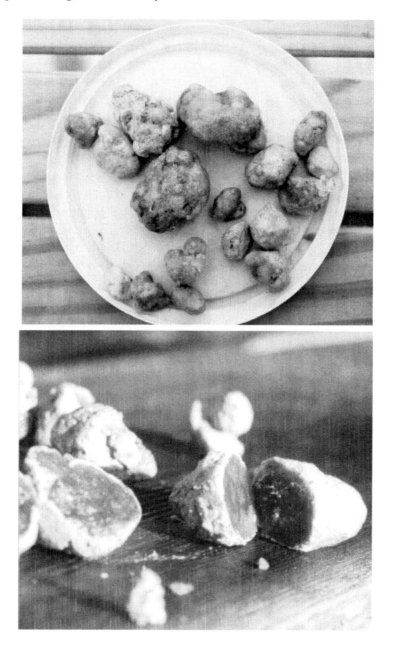

Figures 13c: Calcified and semicalcified gallstones (cut in halves)

As long as there are still a few small stones traveling from some of the thousands of small bile ducts to any of the hundreds of larger bile ducts, they may combine to form larger stones and produce previously experienced symptoms, such as backache, headache, ear ache, digestive trouble, bloating, irritability, anger, and so forth, although these may be less severe than they were before.

If two consecutive new cleanses no longer produce any stones, which may happen after 6 to 8 flushes (in severe cases it may take 10 to 12 or more), your liver can be considered "stone-free." Nevertheless, it is recommended that you repeat the liver flush every six to eight months. Each flush will give a further boost to the liver and take care of any toxins or new stones that may have accumulated in the meantime.

Caution: Never cleanse when you are suffering an acute illness, even if it is just a simple cold. If you suffer from a chronic illness, however, cleansing your liver may be the best thing you can do for yourself.

Important! Please read carefully:

The liver flush is one of the most invaluable and effective methods to regain your health. There are no risks involved if you follow all the directions to the letter. Please take the next cautionary note very seriously. There are many people who have used a liver flush recipe that they received from friends or through the Internet, and they suffered unnecessary complications. They did not have complete knowledge of the procedure and the way it works, believing that just expelling the stones from the liver and gallbladder was sufficient.

It is likely that, on their way out, some gallstones will be caught in the colon. They can quickly be removed through colonic irrigation. This should ideally be done on the second or third day after the liver flush. If gallstones remain in the colon, they can cause irritation, infection, headaches, abdominal discomfort, thyroid problems, and so on. These stones can eventually become a source of toxemia in the body. If colonics are not available where you live, you can take a coffee enema followed by a water enema, or else, do 2 or 3 consecutive water enemas. Still, this may not guarantee that all the remaining stones will be removed. There is no real substitute for colonic irrigation when it comes to liver flushing. Doing a colema-board enema, though, is the closest you can attain to a professional colonic. If you settle for anything less than a colonic irrigation or colema enema, mix one level teaspoon of Epsom salts with one glass of warm water and drink it first thing in the morning on the day of any other chosen colon cleanse following the liver flush. (To acquire a colema-board, see *Product Information* at the end of the book.)

On the importance of colon and kidney cleansing:

Although the liver flush on its own can produce truly amazing results, it should ideally be done *following* a colon and kidney cleanse. Cleansing the colon (see also section on *Preparation*) ensures that the expelled gallstones are easily removed from the large intestine. Cleansing the kidneys makes certain that toxins coming out of the liver during the liver flush do not put any burden on these vital organs of elimination. However, if you have never had kidney trouble, kidney stones, or a bladder infection, you may go ahead with the *colon cleanse—liver flush—colon cleanse sequence*. Nevertheless, make certain that you cleanse the kidneys at a later stage. You should do a kidney cleanse some time after the first 2 to 4 liver flushes and, again, after your liver has been completely cleaned out (see also *The Kidney Cleanse"* in Chapter 5). Instead, you may drink a cup of kidney tea (see "Kidney Cleanse" recipe) for 2 to 3 days after each liver flush. Follow the same directions given for the preparation of the main kidney cleanse. The kidney and liver flushes can be combined, but be sure to avoid drinking the kidney tea on the day of the actual liver flush.

People whose colon is severely congested, or who have a history of constipation, should consider doing at least 2 or 3 colon cleanses before their first liver flush. Moreover, to reemphasize, it is very important that you cleanse your colon within three days of completing each liver flush. Removing gallstones from the liver and gallbladder may leave some of the stones and other toxic residues in the colon. It is essential for your health to clear them out.

A note on drinking water during the cleanse

To reiterate, you may drink water at any time during the liver cleanse, except right after and before taking Epsom salts (allow about 20 minutes). Also, avoid drinking water from 9:30 p.m. until 2 a.m. (if you happen to wake up). Apart from that, you can drink water whenever you are thirsty.

Having Difficulties with the Flush?

Intolerance to Apple Juice

If you cannot tolerate apple juice (or apples) for some reason, you may substitute the following herbs: *gold coin grass* and *bupleurum.* The herbs are made into a tincture and sold as *Gold Coin Grass* (GCG), 8.5 oz. (See *Product Information* at the end of the book.)

Malic acid does exceptionally well at dissolving some of the stagnant bile and making the stones softer. (See details on *malic acid* below.) Cranberry juice also contains malic acid and can be used instead of apple juice. (See below.)

The aforementioned herbs are also effective in softening gallstones and, therefore, can be used as a preparatory step for the liver flush, although it may take a little longer than with using apple or cranberry juice. The proper dosage for the tincture is 1 tablespoonful once daily on an empty stomach, about 30 minutes before breakfast. Keep this regimen for 8 to 9 days before the day of the liver flush.

Intolerance to Epsom Salts

If you are allergic to Epsom salts or just cannot tolerate them, you may use magnesium citrate instead (although it is not quite as effective as Epsom salts). Magnesium citrate is readily available at most drugstores.

Intolerance to Olive Oil

If you are allergic to olive oil or cannot tolerate it, you may use clear macadamia oil, expeller-pressed or cold-pressed grape seed oil, sunflower oil, or other expeller-pressed oils instead. Don't use canola, soy oil, or similar processed oils. (For more information on healthy and harmful oils and fats please refer to the author's book *Timeless Secrets of Health and Rejuvenation.*) Please note that extra virgin olive oil still appears to be the most effective oil for liver cleansing.

You Suffer from Gallbladder Disease or Don't Have a Gallbladder

If you suffer from gallbladder disease or your gallbladder has already been removed, you may need to take cranberry juice or gold coin grass for 2 to 3 weeks (approximately a 1-bottle supply) before liver cleansing. For details, see the previous and following sections.

As a general recommendation, you may also need to consider taking a bile supplement. Most bile supplements contain ox bile. Without a gallbladder, you may never again obtain the right amount of bile needed for the proper digestion of food. If you develop symptoms of diarrhea, lower the dosage or discontinue it. Consult with your health practitioner about which product may be the most suitable for you.

People Who Should Not Use Apple Juice

Some people may have difficulty drinking apple juice in the large quantities required for the liver flush. These include those who suffer from diabetes, hypoglycemia, and yeast infection (*Candida*), cancer, and stomach ulcers.

In any cases of this kind, you may replace apple juice with *malic acid* in powdered form. Avoid malic acid capsules, especially if they contain other ingredients. It is best if the malic acid is properly dissolved before ingesting it. The preparation period is the same as for the apple juice regimen, except that ½ to 1 teaspoon of malic acid, taken with 32 ounces of room-temperature water (or more if it tastes too acidic for you), substitute for the 32 ounces of apple juice per day. Drink this solution in small amounts throughout the day. Food-grade malic acid powder (not mixed with magnesium or other ingredients) is very inexpensive and can be purchased over the Internet or from some natural health food stores. All wineries use malic acid to produce wine. (See *Product Information* at the end of the book.)

Cranberry juice also contains much malic acid and can be used for the preparation period (4 ounces of juice mixed with 4 ounces water, 4 times per day for 6 days). It can also be combined with apple juice. There is added benefit if some cranberry juice is used each day for two or three weeks before liver cleansing.

Another alternative is gold coin grass. Use the same directions as given for those who are intolerant to apple juice. You may try malic acid or cranberry juice during one flush and gold coin grass during the next, to see which works best for you.

A fourth alternative is apple cider vinegar: mix 1 to 2 tablespoons in a glass of water and drink 4 servings per day, for 6 days. However, if Candida is an issue, be aware that vinegar may cause a flare-up of the condition.

Headache or Nausea During the Days Following Liver Flushing

In most cases of headache or nausea in the days after a liver flush, it occurs when the directions have not been followed carefully. (See above section.) However, on some rare occasions, gallstones may continue to pass out of the liver after completing a liver flush. Some toxins released by these stones can enter the circulatory system and cause discomfort. In such a case, it may be helpful to drink about 4 ounces of apple juice for 7 consecutive days, or for as long as the discomfort lasts, following the liver flush. It is best to drink the apple juice at least ½ hour before breakfast. In addition, a repeat colon cleanse may be necessary to clear out any of the late-coming stones. The tissue-cleansing method (ionized water), as mentioned above, also helps to remove the circulating toxins. If you place a small piece of fresh ginger into the thermos flask, drinking this water will quickly stop the nausea. Drinking 2 to 3 cups of chamomile tea per day also helps to calm the digestive tract and the nervous system. Chamomile is also a good "stone-breaker" of calcified stones.

Feeling Sick During the Flush

If you have properly followed all the directions given in the outlined procedure, but still feel sick sometime during the actual liver flush, please do not feel alarmed that something is wrong. Although it occurs rarely, a person may vomit or feel nauseated during the night. This happens when the gallbladder ejects bile and gallstones with such force that bile forces the oil back into the stomach. When the oil, combined with some bile, returns to the stomach, you are likely to feel sick. In such an instance, you may be able to feel the expulsion of stones. It will not be a sharp pain, just a mild contraction.

During one of my 12 liver flushes, I spent a miserable night. But, despite throwing up most of the oil mixture, this flush was just as successful as all the others I had done. By the time I vomited, the oil had already done its job; that is, it prompted the release of gallstones. If this happens to you, remember that this is only one night of discomfort. Recovery from conventional gallbladder surgery may take many weeks or months. Surgery may also lead to major pain and suffering in the years to come.

The Liver Flush Did Not Deliver the Expected Results

In some cases, albeit very rarely, the liver flush does not produce the results you expect. The following are the two main reasons, and their remedies, for such difficulties:

1. It is likely that severe congestion in your liver's bile ducts, due to extremely dense structures of stones, has prevented the apple juice from softening them sufficiently during the first cleansing attempt. In some individuals, it may take as many as 2 or 3 liver flushes before the stones start coming out.

Chanca piedra, also known as "stone-breaker," can help prepare your liver and gallbladder for a more efficient release of stones, especially if you have calcified stones in the gallbladder. Take 20 drops of chanca piedra extract (see *Product Information* at the end of the book) in a glass of water, 3 times daily for at least 2 to 3 weeks before your next flush. Enteric peppermint oil, taken in capsule form, is also very useful in dissolving calcified gallstones or reducing their size. It may not be easy to find it in pure form, though. It is often mixed with other ingredients, which can reduce its effectiveness.

Drinking 2 to 3 cups of chamomile tea per day also helps to dissolve calcified stones.

Another useful method to help support the liver and gallbladder during the flush, and to encourage the release of more stones, is to soak a piece of flannel with heated apple cider vinegar and apply it to the liver/gallbladder area during the 20 to 30-minute period of lying still. Some people have found increased benefits from doing this using warm castor oil instead.

The herbs *Chinese gentian* and *bupleurum,* help to break up some of the congestion and can, thereby, prepare your liver for a more successful flush. These herbs are prepared as a tincture. They are more commonly known as Chinese Bitters. (See *Product Information* at the end of the book.) The proper dosage for this tincture is ½ to 1 teaspoonful once daily on an empty stomach, about 30 minutes before breakfast. This regimen should be followed for three weeks before drinking the apple juice (or using the other alternatives discussed in the previous section). Any unpleasant cleansing reactions usually disappear after 3 to 6 days; they can be minimized by following the tissue-cleansing method of using hot, ionized water and by keeping the colon clean with capsules of oxyflush, oxypowder, colosan, a colema, or an enema (see Chapter 5).

Another method is to drink 3 tablespoons of undiluted, unsweetened lemon juice, 15 to 30 minutes before breakfast daily for one week. This stimulates the gallbladder and makes it ready for a more successful liver flush.

2. You may not have followed the directions properly. Leaving out any one item from the procedure, or altering the dosages or timing of the steps laid out, may prevent you from obtaining the full results. In quite a few people, the liver flush does not work at all unless the large intestine has been cleansed first. The backup of waste and gases cuts down adequate bile secretion and prevents the oil mixture from moving easily through the GI tract. In people who are severely constipated, the gallbladder may barely open up during the liver flush. The best time for a colonic irrigation or an alternative colon cleansing method is the day of the actual liver flush.

Chapter 5

Simple Guidelines to Avoid Gallstones

Once you have eliminated all your gallstones through a series of liver flushes, there are a number of healthful practices you can easily apply that will help your liver to remain permanently clear of stones.

1. Flush Your Liver Twice a Year

I highly recommend that you cleanse your liver twice a year. The best date for a liver flush is about 10 days before or 10 days after a seasonal change. For example, begin the liver flush regimen around March 11 or 31, or June 11 or 30. Repeat the flush 6 months later. When the seasons change, the body also undergoes major physiological changes and is more inclined to release accumulated toxins and waste matter (as seen in an increased incidence of head colds or the flu). Since the immune system is naturally weaker during those 20 days of seasonal adjustment, cleansing the liver supports it greatly in its effort to keep the rest of the body healthy.

2. Keep Your Colon Clean

A weak, irritated, and congested large intestine becomes a breeding place for bacteria that are simply doing their job—decomposing potentially hazardous waste material. As a side effect of their life-saving activities, the microbes produce poisonous substances. Some of these toxins produced by the bacteria enter the blood, which sends them straight to the liver. Constant exposure of the liver cells to these toxins impairs their performance and reduces bile secretion. This leads to a further disruption of digestive functions.

When you eat highly processed foods that have been stripped of most nutrients and natural fiber, the colon has difficulty moving the food mass, or "chyme," along. Processed foods tend to make for a dry, hard, or sticky chyme that passes only with difficulty through the intestinal tract. Normally, the muscles wrapped around the colon can easily squeeze and push fibrous, bulky chyme along, but they struggle greatly dealing with gooey, sticky chyme that is devoid of fiber. When chyme sits too long in the colon, it becomes harder and drier. If that were the only thing that happened—chyme turning into hard, dry feces—we would only need to worry about constipation (from which millions of Americans suffer) and taking laxatives. But there is more to it. After the chyme is plastered onto the walls of the colon, it will undergo biochemical changes and do the following things. It will:

➢ Ferment or putrefy, thereby becoming a breeding ground for parasites and pathogens as well as a storehouse for toxic chemicals. These can pollute the blood and lymph and, thereby, gradually poison the body.
➢ Form a barrier that prevents the colon from interacting with the chyme and absorbing nutrients from it..
➢ Restrict peristaltic movement by the colon walls, making it difficult for the colon to rhythmically contract in order to force the chyme along its way.

How well could you do your job if you were covered with thick sludge? The following are some of the symptoms that may occur as a result of colon dysfunction:

- Lower back pain
- Neck and shoulder pain
- Pain in the lower and upper arms
- Skin problems
- Brain fog (difficulty concentrating)
- Fatigue or sluggishness
- Colds and flu
- Constipation or diarrhea
- Flatulence/gas or bloating

- Crohn's disease
- Ulcerative colitis
- Colitis/irritable bowel syndrome (IBS)
- Diverticulitis/diverticulosis
- Leaky gut syndrome
- Pain in the lower part of the stomach (especially on the left side)

The large intestine absorbs minerals and water. When the membrane of the large intestine is impacted with plaque, it cannot assimilate and absorb minerals (as well as some vitamins). A congested colon causes nutrient-deficiency diseases, regardless of how many supplements a person takes. Most health problems are, in fact, deficiency disorders. They arise when certain parts of the body suffer malnourishment; particularly of minerals (see also *5. Take Ionic Essential Minerals*" in this chapter).

The following are a number of colon-cleansing methods that I recommend in combination with liver flushes:

1. Keeping the colon clean through *colonic irrigation,* for example, is an effective preventive method to safeguard the liver against toxins generated in the large intestine. Colonic irrigation, also known as *colon hydrotherapy,* is perhaps one of the more effective colon therapies. A 30- to 50-minute session can eliminate large amounts of trapped waste that may have taken you many years to accumulate. During a colonic session, the therapist uses a total of 3 to 6 quarts of distilled or purified water to gently cleanse your colon. Through gentle abdominal massage, old deposits of *mucoid fecal matter* are loosened, detached from the colon wall, and subsequently removed with the water.

Colonics tend to have a "relieving" effect. You will usually experience a feeling of lightness, cleanness, and increased clarity of mind following a colonic. However, during the procedure itself, you may feel slight discomfort from time to time, whenever larger quantities of toxic waste detach themselves from the intestinal walls and move toward the rectum.

During the procedure, rubber tubing carries water into the colon and waste out of the colon. The released waste material can be seen floating through a tube, showing the type and quantity of waste eliminated.

Once the colon has been thoroughly cleansed through 2, 3, or more colonics, thereafter diet, exercise, or other health programs are likely to be much more effective. It is estimated that 80 percent of all immune tissue resides in the intestines. Therefore, cleansing the colon from immune-suppressive toxic waste and removing gallstones from the liver can make all the difference in the treatment of cancer, heart disease, AIDS, or other serious illnesses.

Colonic irrigation is a safe and hygienic system for cleansing the colon. Those who have never experienced a colonic, or who have a vested interest in dissuading others from having one, are the most likely people to raise safety concerns about colonics.

2. If you do not have access to a colon therapist, you may greatly benefit from using a *colema board* (see *Product Information* at the end of the book) as a second-best choice. The colema board allows you to clean your colon in the comfort of your own home. The colema is a do-it-yourself enema treatment that is easy to learn and perform.

3. *Colosan* is a blend of various oxides of magnesium designed to gently release oxygen into the digestive tract for cleansing it. Colosan is a powder that you either mix with water and chase down with citrus juice or take in capsule form, which is more convenient. Colosan releases large amounts of oxygen in the intestinal tract, thereby eliminating old fecal material as well as parasites and hardened mucus (see *Product Information*). Oxypowder is a similar product that works just as well.

4. Another method of cleansing, which uses Epsom salts, cleanses not only the colon but also the small intestine. This may become necessary if you have major difficulties absorbing food, have repeated kidney/bladder congestion, experience severe constipation, or are simply unable to do a colonic. For 3 weeks, add 1 teaspoon of oral Epsom salts (magnesium sulfate) to 1 glass of warm water and drink this first thing in the morning. This oral enema flushes your entire digestive tract and colon, from top to bottom, usually within an hour, prompting you to eliminate several times. It clears out even some of the plaque and debris from the intestinal walls, along with the parasites that have been living there. Expect the stools to be watery for as long as there is intestinal waste to be disposed of. Stools adopt a more normal shape and consistency once the entire intestinal tract is clean. This treatment can be done 2 to 3 times per year. Expect some cramps or gas formation, at times, while on this cleanse (a result of releasing toxins). Your tongue may become white-coated and be thicker than normal. This indicates increased intestinal cleansing. Epsom salts are not tolerated by everyone.

5. Castor oil is a traditionally used, excellent remedy to clear waste material from the intestines. It is less irritating than Epsom salts and has no side effects other than normal cleansing reactions. Take 1 to 3 teaspoons of castor oil in 1/3 glass of warm water on an empty stomach in the morning or before going to sleep at night (depending on which works better for you). It is a very beneficial treatment for stubborn cases of constipation. It can also be given to children (in smaller dosages). Although it is not recommended to replace Epsom salts with any other intestinal cleanser during the liver flush, in case of an allergy to Epsom salts magnesium citrate or castor oil may be used instead.

6. Aloe vera juice is another effective way to cleanse the GI tract. However, it is not a replacement for the colonics or colemas before and after a liver flush. Aloe vera has both nourishing and cleansing effects. One tablespoon of aloe vera juice, diluted with a little water, before meals or at least once in the morning before breakfast, helps to break down old deposits of waste and bring basic nutrients to cells and tissues. Those who feel their liver is still releasing many toxins several days after a liver flush may greatly benefit from drinking aloe vera juice.

Aloe vera has been found to be effective in almost every illness, including cancer, heart disease, and AIDS. It is helpful for all kinds of allergies, skin diseases, blood disorders, arthritis, infections, Candida, cysts, diabetes, eye problems, digestive problems, ulcers, liver diseases, hemorrhoids, high blood pressure, kidney stones, and strokes, to name a few. Aloe vera contains over 200 nutrients, including the vitamins B1, B2, B3, B6, C, E, and folic acid; iron, calcium, magnesium, zinc, manganese, copper, barium, sulphate; 18 amino acids; important enzymes; glycosides; and polysaccharides, among others. Make certain you purchase only pure, undiluted aloe vera, available in health food stores. One of the best brands is produced by the company *Lily of the Desert* (in Denton, Texas). It is made of 99.7 percent organic aloe vera juice, with no water added.

Caution: With regular drinking of aloe vera juice, diabetics may improve the ability of their pancreas to produce more of its own insulin. Therefore, diabetics should consult their physician to monitor their need for extra insulin, since too much insulin is dangerous. Many diabetics report a reduction in the amount of insulin required. Make certain you purchase only undiluted aloe vera juice.

If you experience diarrhea after taking aloe vera juice, try reducing the dosage. Not everyone benefits from aloe vera.

7. Small enema treatments (in comparison to colonics or colemas) involve the introduction of liquids into the rectum (usually, that is as far as they reach) for the purpose of cleansing and nourishment. An enema has an immediate effect on nearly all parts of the body. It alleviates constipation, distension, chronic fever, the common cold, headaches, sexual disorders, kidney stones, pain in the heart area, vomiting, low backache, stiffness and pain in the neck and shoulders, nervous disorders, hyperacidity, and tiredness. Moreover, disorders such as arthritis, rheumatism, sciatica, and gout may greatly benefit from an enema. Recommended liquids include filtered water, certain herbal teas, coffee, or oil. (For a detailed description of each enema type, see my book, *Timeless Secrets of Health and Rejuvenation.*)

3. The Kidney Cleanse

If the presence of gallstones in the liver, or any other situation, has led to the development of sand, grease, or stones in the kidneys or urinary bladder, you may also need to cleanse your kidneys. The kidneys are extremely delicate, blood-filtering organs that congest easily because of dehydration, poor diet, weak digestion, stress, and an irregular lifestyle. The main causes of congestion in the kidneys are kidney stones. Most kidney grease/crystals/stones, however, are too small to be detected through modern diagnostic technology, including ultrasounds or x-rays. They are often called "silent" stones and do not seem to bother people much. When they grow larger, though, they can cause considerable distress and damage to the kidneys and the rest of the body. To prevent kidney problems and kidney-related diseases, it is best to eliminate kidney stones before they can cause a crisis. You can easily detect the presence of sand or stones in the kidneys by pulling the skin under your eyes sideways toward the cheekbones. Any irregular bumps, protrusions, red or white pimples, or discoloration of the skin indicates the presence of kidney sand or kidney stones.

The following herbs, when taken daily for a period of twenty to thirty days, can help to dissolve and eliminate all types of kidney stones, including uric acid, oxalic acid, phosphate, and amino acid stones. If you have a history of kidney stones, you may need to repeat this cleanse a few times, at intervals of six weeks.

Ingredients:

Marjoram (1 oz.)
Cat's claw (1 oz.)
Comfrey root (1 oz.)
Fennel seed (2 oz.)
Chicory herb (2 oz.)

Uva ursi (2 oz.)
Hydrangea root (2 oz.)
Gravel root (2 oz.)
Marshmallow root (2 oz.)
Golden rod herb (2 oz.)

Directions:

Take 1 ounce each of the first three herbs and 2 ounces each of the rest of the herbs, and thoroughly mix them together. Keep them in an airtight container. You may put them in the refrigerator. Before bedtime, soak 3 tablespoons of the mixture in 2 cups of water, cover it, and leave it covered overnight. The following morning, bring the concoction to a boil; then strain it. If you forget to soak the herbs in the evening, boil the mixture in the morning, and let it simmer for 5 to 10 minutes before straining.

Drink a few sips at a time in 6 to 8 portions throughout the day. This tea does not need to be taken warm or hot, but do not refrigerate it. Also, *do not* add sugar or sweeteners! Leave at least one hour after eating before taking your next sips.

Repeat this procedure for twenty days. If you experience discomfort or stiffness in the area of the lower back, this is because mineral crystals from kidney stones are passing through the ureter ducts of the urinary system. Any strong smell and darkening of the urine at the beginning of or during the kidney cleanse indicates a major release of toxins from the kidneys. Normally, though, the release is gradual and does not significantly change the color or texture of the urine. **Important***:* Support the kidneys during the cleanse by drinking extra amounts of water, a minimum of six and a maximum of eight glasses per day, unless the color of the urine is dark-yellow (in which case you will need to drink more than that amount).

During the cleanse, try to avoid consuming animal products, including meat, dairy foods (except butter), fish, eggs, tea, coffee, alcohol, carbonated beverages, chocolate, and any other foods or drinks that contain preservatives, artificial sweeteners, coloring agents, and the like. In addition to drinking this kidney tea each day, if convenient, you may also chew on a small piece of rind from an organic lemon on the left side of your mouth and a small piece of carrot on the right side of your mouth 30 to 40 times each. This stimulates kidney functions. Be sure to allow at least half an hour between chewing cycles.

If you are doing liver flushes, make certain that you do a kidney cleanse after every three or four liver flushes.

In addition, those suffering from large kidney stones may benefit from drinking the juice of one to two lemons (diluted with water) per day for about ten to fourteen days. After that, drink the juice of half a lemon per day indefinitely.

4. Drink Ionized Water Frequently

The sipping of hot ionized water has a profound cleansing effect on all the tissues of the body. It helps reduce overall toxicity, improves circulatory functions, and balances bile. When you boil water for 15 to 20 minutes, it becomes thinner (its molecule clusters are reduced from the normal number of about 10,000 to one or two clusters), and it is charged and saturated with negative oxygen ions (hydroxide, OH^-). When you take frequent sips of this water throughout the day, it begins to systematically cleanse the tissues of the body and help rid them of certain positively charged ions (those associated with harmful acids and toxins).

Most toxins and waste materials carry a positive charge and, thus, naturally tend to attach themselves to the body, which is negatively charged overall. As the negative oxygen ions enter the body with the ingested water, they are attracted to the positively charged toxic material. This neutralizes waste and toxins, turning them into fluid matter that the body can remove easily. For the first couple of days or even weeks of cleansing your body tissues in this way, your tongue may take on a white or yellow coating, an indication that the body is clearing out a lot of toxic waste. If you have excessive body weight, this cleansing method can help you shed many pounds of body waste in a short period of time, without the side effects that normally accompany sudden weight loss.

Directions: Boil water for 15 to 20 minutes and pour it into a thermos. Stainless steel thermoses are fine. The thermos keeps the water hot and ionized throughout the day. Take one or two sips every half hour all day long, and drink it as hot as you would sip tea. You may use this method anytime you do not feel well, have the need for decongesting, wish to keep the blood thin, or simply want to feel more energetic and clear. Some people drink ionized water for a certain duration, such as three to four weeks; others do it ongoing.

The oxygen ions are generated through the bubbling effect of boiling water, similar to water falling on the ground in a waterfall or breaking against the seashore. In the thermos, the water will stay ionized for up to 12 hours or for as long as it remains hot. The total amount of water you need to boil to give you enough hot, ionized water for one day would be about 20 to 24 ounces. This specially prepared water should not substitute for normal drinking water. It doesn't hydrate the cells like normal water does; the body uses it to only cleanse the tissues.

5. Take Ionic Essential Minerals

Your body is like "living soil." If it has sufficient minerals and trace elements to work with, it is able to nurture you and produce everything you need to live and grow. These essential materials, however, can easily become depleted when you do not get enough of them from the food you eat. Centuries of constant use of the same agricultural fields have led to foods that are highly nutrient-deficient. The situation worsened with the onset of chemical fertilizers, which force crops to grow more rapidly without regard for nutrient availability. When minerals and trace elements run low in the body, important functions can no longer be sustained, or they become subdued. Disease is generally accompanied by a lack of one or more of these important substances.

Because of the unnatural situation of mineral depletion in our soil today and, therefore, in our bodies, it may be useful to supplement with minerals. The crucial question is whether the minerals sold in nutrition stores or pharmacies are capable of replenishing the mineral supply to the cells of the body. The answer is, "Highly unlikely!"

Minerals are commonly made available in three basic forms: capsules, tablets, and colloidal mineral water. Before the depletion of soils, plant foods were our ideal mineral provider. When a plant grows in a healthy soil environment, it absorbs existing colloidal minerals and changes them into ionic, eater-soluble form. The ionic minerals are an angstrom in size, whereas the colloidal minerals, also known as inorganic, metallic minerals, are about 10,000 times larger (micron-size). Ionic, water-soluble plant minerals are absorbed readily by body cells. In contrast, colloidal particles packed into complex compounds, and delivered in pill form, stand less than a 1 percent chance of absorption. The minerals found in colloidal mineral waters are not absorbed any better. They are not water-soluble, but simply suspended between water molecules.

Common colloidal particles, such as the compounds calcium carbonate and zinc picolinate, tend to get caught in the bloodstream and are subsequently deposited in various parts of the body. In the form of deposits, they can cause major mechanical, structural, and functional damage. Many health problems today, including osteoporosis, heart disease, cancer, arthritis, brain disorders, kidney stones, gallstones, and so on, are the direct result of ingesting such metallic minerals.

Fortunately, there is a very efficient way to obtain minerals in the size of, and with the characteristics of, plant minerals. When vaporized in a vacuum chamber (without oxygen), minerals are prevented from oxidizing and forming into complex states. Once vaporized, the minerals can be combined with purified water and be made readily available to the cells of the body. One company located in Minnesota has managed to create a delivery process capable of converting colloids into 99.9 percent water-soluble, ionic minerals. The company, Eniva, makes these minerals available via distributorship (see *Product Information* at the end of the book).[28] More companies now offer similar ionic minerals; you can easily locate them on the Internet.

6. Drinking Enough Water

To produce the right amount of bile each day (1–1½ quarts), which the body requires for proper digestion of food, the liver needs plenty of water. In addition, the body uses up a lot of water to maintain normal blood volume, hydrate the cells and connective tissues, cleanse out toxins, and carry out literally thousands of other functions. Since the body cannot store water the way it stores fat, it is dependent on regular, sufficient water intake.

To maintain proper bile production and bile consistency, as well as balanced blood values, you need to drink about six to eight glasses of water each day. The most important time to drink water is right after getting up: First, drink one glass of warm water to make it easier for the kidneys to dilute and excrete urine formed during the night. This is of great importance because urine is highly concentrated in the morning; if it is not diluted properly, urinary waste products may settle in both the kidneys and the

---

[28] The author recommends Eniva minerals to his clients as a method of prevention of illness and to promote good health. (**Note:** To order any products from Eniva (www.eniva.com), you require a sponsor name and ID. You may use the name and ID of the author, Andreas Moritz, #13462.)

urinary bladder. Second, drink another glass of warm water to which you can add the juice of 1 slice up to ½ of a fresh lemon and 1 teaspoon of raw honey. This helps to cleanse the GI tract.

Other important times for drinking a glass of water (not chilled) are about ½ hour before and 2½ hours after meals. These are the times when a well-hydrated body would naturally signal thirst. Having enough water available at those times ensures that the blood, bile, and lymph remain sufficiently fluid to conduct their respective activities in the body. Since hunger and thirst signals use the same hormonal alert system in the body, if you happen to feel "hungry" during those times, it is more likely that you are actually running out of water. Therefore, it is best to drink a glass of room temperature or warm water first and then see whether your hunger has subsided or not.

If you suffer from high blood pressure and use medicinal drugs for this condition, make sure you have your blood pressure monitored regularly. With an increase in your water consumption, your blood pressure may return to normal within a relatively short period of time. This would make the intake of medication obsolete and even harmful. By drinking enough water, you may also start to lose weight if you are overweight, or gain weight if you are underweight.

It is equally important to choose a water treatment system that gives you fresh, healthy water. The H_2O water treatment system is, for example, is very efficient and health-promoting, but it is also quite expensive. Its unique technology even removes pesticides and herbicides from the water and leaves your drinking, shower, and pool water as fresh and clean as pure mountain water.

The H_2O Concept 2000 uses electrical impulses to break calcium bicarbonate and magnesium bicarbonate, salts that are the major causes of hard water, into calcium carbonate and magnesium carbonate with the by-product being carbon dioxide (CO_2). The CO_2 is dispelled at the faucet in minuscule amounts. Calcium carbonate and magnesium carbonate are the soluble forms of these two minerals. In their soluble state, these minerals compounds cannot adhere to the inner surfaces of pipes, water heaters coils, glass surfaces, faucets, and so forth. Thus, mineral buildup and the formation of scale are impossible. The H_2O Concept 2000 will also significantly reduce any existing scale over time. This gives all water-using appliances in your home a longer and more efficient life span. Although quite pricey at the beginning, this water treatment system saves you money in the end. It is also virtually maintenance-free. Quite a few similar filters are now available, some cheaper, others even more expensive. I personally use a *Puritec* whole house water filter, which is similar to the H_2O Concept 2000. When you choose a water treatment system, make sure it has the mixed-media **KDF/GAC** filtration technology.

Quite affordable, yet still very effective, and excellent for people who not only are interested in proper hydration but also want to cleanse the body from toxins, are water ionizers. These are widely available on the Internet.

The most commonly used methods to remove chlorine and numerous other contaminants from your drinking water (and possibly shower water) are filtration and reverse osmosis. Although these systems can also be pricey, they are still an affordable option if you consider the cost of suffering through a bout of cancer. To help replenish some of the minerals lost when using these two types of systems, add a few grains of uncooked basmati rice to the water jug or bottle (avoid plastic containers) and leave the rice in the jar for up to a month at a time. Adding a pinch of or unrefined sea salt to a glass of water also helps to give you the lost minerals back.

Distilled water, which is the closest to natural rainwater, is excellent for hydrating the body cells, but, unlike rainwater, it is lifeless. Adding 3 to four 4 of uncooked basmati rice to 1 gallon of distilled water gives it minerals and vitamins (or else use the sea salt option), and exposing the water to direct sunlight or placing a clear quartz crystal in the water for an hour helps to restore its vitality. The only machine I know of that produces healthy, energized distilled water is the "Crystal Clear electron water/air machine™," developed by John Ellis (johnellis.com). Its water even eliminates the smell in waste lagoons and septic systems (it kills only harmful bacteria).

Of course, the old-fashioned method of boiling your drinking water for several minutes causes any chlorine to evaporate.

Another inexpensive way to get rid of most chlorine in water is to use vitamin C. One gram of vitamin C will neutralize 1ppm (part per million) of chlorine in 100 gallons of water. This is particularly useful if you want to lie in the bathtub without suffering the irritating effects of chlorine on your skin and in your lungs.

Prill beads are another, far less expensive, form of water treatment. Although they cannot replace a water filter, they still cleanse your drinking water and make it "thinner." This has a positive effect on the blood, lymph, and basic cellular processes. Prill beads are available on the Internet (see suppliers lists at the end of the book). I can attest to the good taste of the water, its "thinness," and its excellent hydrating and cleansing effects.

Yet another good water treatment is Molecular Resonance Effect Technology (MRET)—a device that alters the molecular organizational state of water and other liquid substances. MRET Water has many special properties that make it ideal to help the body to increase its quota of structured water. MRET-activated water closely resembles cellular water in the body and hence is bioavailable. MRET Water is produced by means of a nonchemical biosafe process of water activation. During this process, a subtle, low-frequency electromagnetic field is imprinted into the water. It is similar to the earth's geomagnetic field found in special healing springs. I have tested the basic MRET and found it to be very beneficial, although it requires separate filtering. It is widely available on the Internet. NIKKEN also makes an excellent water treatment system.

7. Cut Down on Alcohol

Alcohol is liquefied, refined sugar and is highly acid-forming. Therefore, it has a strong mineral-depleting effect in the body. The organ most affected by alcohol is the liver. If a generally healthy person drinks two glasses of wine within one hour, the liver is not able to detoxify all the alcohol. Much of it is converted into fatty deposits and, eventually, gallstones in the liver. If the liver and gallbladder have already accumulated a number of gallstones, alcohol consumption will make these stones grow faster and cause them to become more plentiful.

Like coffee or tea, alcohol has a strongly dehydrating effect. It reduces the water content of the body's cells, blood, lymph, and bile, thus impairing blood circulation and the elimination of waste products. The effects of a dehydrated central nervous system are delirium, blurred vision, a loss of memory and orientation, and slow reaction time, all of which we generally refer to as a "hangover." Under the influence of alcohol and the dehydration it causes, the nervous and immune systems go into depression. This leads to a slowing of the digestive, metabolic, and hormonal processes in the body. All of this promotes the development of even more gallstones in the liver and gallbladder.

It is best for those who have had a history of gallstones to avoid alcohol altogether. Many of my clients who stopped drinking any kind of alcohol, including beer and wine, spontaneously recovered from such problems as panic attacks, arrhythmia, respiratory problems, various heart conditions, sleeping disorders, gallbladder attacks, pancreatic infections, prostate enlargement, colitis, and other inflammatory diseases. If you suffer from any disease at all, it is best to stay away from all dehydrating beverages, such as alcohol, coffee, tea, and soda (especially diet drinks). This allows the body to direct all its energy and resources toward healing the affected part or parts of the body.

8. Avoid Overeating

One of the greatest causes of gallstones is *overindulging in food*. Eating more than the stomach can process without suffering indigestion or "fullness" causes the liver to secrete excessive amounts of cholesterol into liver bile. This, in turn, leads to the development of gallstones in the bile ducts. Therefore, one of the most effective methods to prevent gallstones is "undereating."

Eating in moderation and observing an occasional day of "fasting" on just liquids (ideally once per week) both help the digestive system to remain efficient and able to deal with most existing deposits of undigested food. Liquids include vegetable soups, fruit juices, vegetable juices, herbal teas, and water. Leaving the dining table while still a little hungry maintains a healthy desire for good, nutritious foods. Overeating, by contrast, leads to intestinal congestion, the proliferation of destructive bacteria and yeast, and cravings for "energizing," which really means energy-depleting, foods and beverages, such as sugar, sweets, white flour products, potato chips, chocolate, coffee, tea, and soft drinks. All these foods and beverages lead to gallstone formation.

9. Maintain Regular Mealtimes

The body is controlled by numerous circadian rhythms, which regulate the most important functions in the body in accordance with preprogrammed time intervals. Sleep, the secretion of hormones and digestive juices, the elimination of waste, and so on, all follow a specific daily "routine." If these cyclic activities become disrupted more often than they are adhered to, the body becomes imbalanced and cannot fulfill its essential tasks. All tasks are naturally aligned with and dependent on the schedule dictated by the circadian rhythms.

Having regular mealtimes makes it easy for the body to prepare for the production and secretion of the right amounts of digestive juices for each meal. Irregular eating habits, on the other hand, confuse the body. Furthermore, its digestive power becomes depleted by having to adjust to a different mealtime each time you eat. Skipping meals here and there, eating at different times, or eating between meals especially disrupts the cycles of bile production by the liver cells. The result is the formation of gallstones.

By maintaining a regular eating routine, the body's 60 to 100 trillion cells are able to receive their daily ratio of nutrients according to schedule, which helps cell metabolism to be smooth and effective. Many metabolic disorders, such as diabetes or obesity, result from irregular eating habits and can be greatly improved by matching one's eating times with the natural circadian rhythms. It is best to eat the largest meal of the day around midday and only light meals at breakfast (no later than 8:00 a.m.) and dinner (no later than 7:00 p.m.).

10. Eat a Vegetarian/Vegan Diet

Eating a balanced vegetarian/vegan diet is one of the most effective ways to prevent the formation of gallstones, heart disease, and cancer. If you feel you cannot solely live on foods that are of vegetable origin, then at least try to substitute red meat with chicken, rabbit, or turkey for some time. Eventually, you may be able to go fully vegetarian. All forms of animal protein decrease the solubility of bile, which is a major risk factor for gallstones.

You can greatly reduce the risk of developing gallstones by adding more vegetables, salads, fruit, and complex carbohydrates to your diet. Drinking 2 to 3 ounces of fresh carrot juice daily before lunch prevents stones from being formed. Aged cheese, commercial yogurt, and highly processed and refined foods create an imbalanced constitution of bile. Moreover, try to avoid fried and deep-fried foods. Consuming the heated oils (packed with harmful trans fats) used by fast food restaurants are an especially quick way to produce gallstones.

For complete guidelines on how to eat a healthy, life-sustaining diet according to your body type, see *Timeless Secrets of Health and Rejuvenation.*

11. Avoid "Light" Food Products

Several scientific studies show that eating "light foods" actually encourages appetite and overeating, and does **not** reduce weight. Before they were introduced into the human food chain, "light foods" were fed to animals that subsequently began to gain weight faster than normal. The same happened in humans when they started eating these unnatural foods on a regular basis.

The Director of the Framingham Study[29] - William Castelli, M.D., published this astonishing quote in the July 1992 issue of the Archives of Internal Medicine: "At Framingham, we found that the people who ate the most saturated fat, the most cholesterol and the most calories weighed the least, were more physically active and had the lowest serum cholesterol levels."

The more *enzymatic energy* that is contained in food, the faster we feel satisfied and the more efficiently the food is converted into usable energy and bioavailable nutrients. In contrast, eating low-calorie, "light foods" impairs bile secretion, digestion, and

---

[29] The Framingham study is the longest, most expensive, and largest sample-size heart disease study in history.

excretory functions. Elevated levels of blood fat indicate that bile secretions are low, blood vessel walls are thickening, and fats are not being adequately digested and absorbed. Hence, a person with high blood fats actually suffers from a fat deficiency. In direct response to an increased demand for fats in the cells and tissues of the body, a low-fat diet may actually raise cholesterol production in the liver. The side effects of this survival maneuver by the body include the development of gallstones, weight gain, and/or wasting.

Low-fat and other low-calorie diets are damaging to one's health and should be prescribed only, if at all, in acute liver and gallbladder disorders where the digestion and absorption of fat are severely disrupted. After all gallstones are removed and liver functions are normalized, it is necessary to gradually increase fat and calorie consumption to meet the high-energy demands of the human body. The presence of gallstones in the liver and gallbladder impair the body's ability to properly digest fat and other kinds of high-energy food. Even minimal consumption of useless "light foods" interferes with the body's most basic metabolic and hormonal processes if these "foods" are ingested for a period of several years. The result may be serious repercussions for one's health. By eating a diet low in protein, as well as cleansing the liver and gallbladder, normal, balanced fat intake will not put you at risk for developing gallbladder or liver problems.

12. Eat Unrefined Sea Salt

Refined salt has virtually no benefits for the body. On the contrary, it is responsible for causing numerous health problems, including gallstones. The only salt that the body can digest, assimilate, and utilize properly is unrefined, unprocessed sea salt or rock salt. For salt to be useful to the body, it needs to penetrate foods—that is, the moisture of the fruits, vegetables, grains, and legumes must be allowed to dissolve the salt. If salt is used in its dry state, it enters the body in a nonionized form and creates thirst (a sign of being poisoned). It causes further harm because it is not being properly assimilated and utilized. (See Chapter 3.)

You may dissolve a pinch of salt in a small amount of water and add that to fruit or other foods that are not usually cooked. This will aid in the digestion of those items while helping to deacidify the body. Adding a pinch of salt to drinking water generates alkaline properties and provides you with important minerals and trace elements.

It may be worth mentioning that food should taste delicious, but not salty, in and of itself. Pitta and Kapha body types require less salt than does the Vata body type.[30] (To purchase untreated and unrefined sea salt, see *Product Information* at the end of the book.)

Important Functions of Real Salt in the Body:

- Stabilizes irregular heartbeat and regulates blood pressure—in conjunction with water
- Extracts excess acidity from the cells in the body, particularly the brain cells
- Balances sugar levels in the blood, which is particularly important for diabetics
- Is essential for the generation of hydroelectric energy in the cells of the body
- Is vital for the absorption of nutrient components through the intestinal tract
- Is needed to clear the lungs of mucus and sticky phlegm, particularly in those suffering from asthma and cystic fibrosis
- Clears up catarrh and congestion in the sinuses
- Is a strong natural antihistamine
- Can prevent muscle cramps
- Helps prevent excess saliva production; saliva that is flowing out of the mouth during sleep may indicate salt deficiency
- Makes bones firm; 27 percent of the body's salt content is located in the bones; salt deficiency and/or eating refined salt versus real salt are major causes of osteoporosis
- Regulates sleep; acts as a natural hypnotic
- Helps prevent gout and gouty arthritis
- Is vital for maintaining sexuality and libido

---

[30] To determine your Ayurvedic body type, refer to *Timeless Secrets of Health and Rejuvenation.*

- Can prevent varicose veins and spider veins on the legs and thighs
- Supplies the body with over 80 essential mineral elements; refined salt, such as the common table salt, has been stripped of all but two of these elements; In addition, refined, commercial salt contains harmful additives, including aluminum silicate, a primary cause of Alzheimer's disease.

13. The Importance of *Ener-Chi Art*

Ener-Chi Art is a unique method of rejuvenation that helps restore a balanced flow of Chi (vital energy) through the organs and systems in the body, within less than one minute. I consider this healing approach to be a profound tool in facilitating a more successful outcome to all other natural healing methods. When Chi flows properly through the cells of the body, the cells can more efficiently remove their metabolic waste products; more readily absorb all the oxygen, water, and nutrients they need; and conduct any necessary repair work more swiftly. The body can restore its health and vitality much more easily when there is constant, unrestricted availability of Chi. Although I consider the liver flush to be one of the most effective tools to help the body return to balanced functioning, by itself it may not be able to restore the body's overall vital energy, as a result of many years of congestion and deterioration. Test results have shown that *Ener-Chi Art* may very well fill this gap.

The use of *Ener-Chi Ionized Stones* is another practical and effective tool to improve one's health and vitality. (For more information on *Ener-Chi Art* and Ionized Stones, see *Other Books, Products, and Services by the Author* at the end of this book.)

14. Getting Enough Sleep

Tiredness precedes any type of disease, whether it is cancer, heart disease, or AIDS. Although impaired liver functions, low immunity, and overeating can also cause fatigue, in most cases it results from a lack of quality sleep, that is, the sleep before midnight.

Some of the most vital processes of purification and rejuvenation in the body are initiated and carried out during the two hours of sleep before midnight. Physiologically, there are two entirely different types of sleep, as verified by brain wave measurements. These are *before-midnight sleep* and *after-midnight sleep.* Sleep that occurs in the two hours before midnight includes deep sleep and it is often referred to as "beauty sleep." Deep sleep occurs for about one hour and generally lasts from 11:00 p.m. to midnight. During deep sleep, you are in a dreamless state of consciousness where oxygen consumption in the body drops by about 8 percent. The rest and relaxation that you gain during this hour of dreamless sleep is nearly three times as deep as you would get from the same amount of sleep after midnight (when oxygen consumption in the body rises again).

Deep sleep hardly ever occurs after midnight. You experience deep sleep only if you go to sleep at least two hours before midnight. If you regularly miss out on deep sleep, your body and mind become overtired and your stress responses become unnaturally high. Stress responses include secretions of the stress hormones *adrenaline, cortisol,* and *cholesterol.* (A part of the cholesterol secreted during a stress response may end up as gallstones.) To keep these artificially derived energy bursts going, you may feel the urge to use such nerve stimulants as cigarettes, coffee, tea, candy, colas, or alcohol. When the body's energy reserves are finally exhausted, chronic fatigue results.

When you feel tired, all of your body''s cells are tired, not just your mind. In fact, your organs, digestive system, nervous system, and the like, will also suffer from a lack of energy and will not be able to function properly. When you are tired, your brain no longer receives adequate amounts of water, glucose, oxygen, and amino acids, which make up its main food supply. This situation can lead to innumerable problems in your mind, body, and behavior.

Doctors at the University of California in San Diego have found that losing a few hours of sleep not only makes you feel tired the next day, but can also affect the immune system, possibly impairing the body's ability to fight infection. Since immunity diminishes with increasing fatigue, your body is unable to defend itself against bacteria, microbes, and viruses and cannot cope with the buildup of toxic substances in the body. Getting enough sleep, therefore, is the most important prerequisite for restoring health to the body and mind. Try to go to sleep before 10:00 p.m. and to rise between 6:00 and 7:00 a.m., or earlier, depending on your sleep requirements. It is best not to use an alarm clock, to allow for a natural phasing out of your sleeping cycles. Removing all gallstones from the liver and gallbladder and getting enough sleep will reduce any tiredness that you may be experiencing during the day. Should the problem continue, the kidneys may need to be cleansed as well. (To dissolve kidney stones, see *The Kidney Cleanse*" in Chapter 5.)

15. Avoid Overworking

Working too hard for too many hours overtaxes the body's energy system. Overworking particularly stresses the liver. To meet the excessive demand for energy in the brain or in other parts of the body, the liver tries to convert as much complex sugar into simple sugars (glucose) as possible. If a shortfall of energy occurs, or if energy supplies run out altogether, the body must take recourse to an emergency stress response, which makes extra energy available, but at the same time disrupts circulatory and immune functions.

The continuous secretion of adrenaline and other stress hormones that occurs in a person who "never stops working" can eventually turn him or her into a *workaholic*. This is a condition in which work becomes the major source of excitement in that person's life. The excitement is provided by the "thrill effect" brought about by the stress hormones.

To avoid exhausting your liver and damaging your immune system, make enough time for yourself. Try to allocate at least one hour each day for meditation, yoga, exercise, listening to music, artistic activities, or being outdoors enjoying nature. The body is not a machine that can run continuously without a break. Overworking the body and mind in any way will eventually demand extra recovery time from an illness. In the long run, overworking as a means to get things done faster, or to earn money more quickly, not only cuts years off one's life but also cuts life off one's years, as the old saying goes.

The liver is designed to provide energy for a certain number of years; overextending this "service" damages or destroys the liver prematurely. Living by a code of moderation with regard to eating, sleeping, and working will enable you to maintain an efficient and vital energy system throughout life. Another old saying recommends that we spend one-third of our life sleeping, one-third working, and one-third enjoying recreational pursuits. This wise formula maintains balance on all levels of life: physical, mental, and spiritual. Overworking upsets this much-needed state of equilibrium among our body, mind, and spirit.

16. Exercise Regularly

Our technological and economic advancement has led to an increasingly sedentary lifestyle, which requires additional forms of physical movement to keep our bodies vital and healthy. Regular exercise helps to increase our capacity to digest food, eliminate physical impurities, balance our emotions, promote firmness and suppleness, and strengthen our ability to deal with stressful situations. When performed in moderation, exercise serves as a great immune stimulant and improves neuromuscular integration in all age groups. Boosting self-confidence and self-esteem are important by-products of exercise that stem from an improved oxygen supply to the cells—not to mention the improvement in self-esteem that comes from losing excess fat, seeing muscle definition, feeling stronger, and generally looking great. All this results in greater well-being, both physically and mentally.

The liver, especially, seems to benefit from aerobic exercise. The increased availability of oxygen during and after exercise greatly improves circulation and enhances the flow of venous blood from the liver toward the heart. A sedentary lifestyle slows this process, causing blood flow in the liver to stagnate. This, in turn, leads to the development of gallstones. For that reason, regular, nonstrenuous exercise can prevent new stones from forming.

By contrast, the physical exertion that results from overexercising leads to the secretion of excessive amounts of stress hormones, leaving the body restless and shaky. When the body is depleted of energy, it is unable to do the repair work that arises from a strenuous workout. Thus, the cardiovascular system is left weak and vulnerable to other stress factors as well. Overexertion can also have a detrimental effect on the thymus gland. Specifically, the thymus gland, which activates *lymphocytes* (immune cells that defend us against disease) and controls energy supplies, may actually shrink in size, causing the body to become agitated and vulnerable to all kinds of health problems. In light of this, it is best to choose a form of exercise that gives you a sense of joy and satisfaction. Whenever you exercise, make certain that you always breathe through your nose and keep your mouth closed, in order to avoid the harmful *"adrenaline breathing."* (Rapid mouth breathing usually occurs during a typical fight-or-flight response and can trigger the release of stress hormones, and it can do the same even without a stress response.) Aerobic exercises are effective and beneficial as long as you maintain nasal breathing (versus mouth breathing). If you run out of breath, slow down or stop exercising. You may resume the exercise once your breathing returns to normal. This simple advice can prevent you from potential harm, such as exhaustion or the production of too much lactic acid that can easily occur from overexercising.

Considering how crucial exercise is for a healthy body and mind, try to exercise every day, even if it is only for 10 minutes. It is important, though, not to exceed 50 percent of your capacity for exercise. The main thing is to avoid becoming fatigued. For example, if you can swim for 30 minutes before getting tired, swim for only 15 minutes. In time, your capacity for exercise will increase. Remember, both excessive exercise and a lack of it weaken the immune system, impair liver functions, and flood the blood with harmful substances.

A simple hand exercise/massage is helpful both to prevent problems and to aid in the treatment of the liver and gallbladder. Massage the outer edge of each hand, near the base of the little finger— massaging out any tenderness there. This stimulates a sluggish liver and gallbladder.

17. Get Regular Exposure to Sunlight

Your body is capable of synthesizing vitamin D (which is actually a hormone rather than a vitamin) through a process whereby the sun's ultraviolet rays interact with a form of cholesterol present in the skin. Regular exposure to sunlight has been shown to regulate cholesterol levels. However, unlike cholesterol-lowering drugs, sunlight does *not* increase cholesterol in the bile, which is a major cause of gallstones. Sunlight has a holistic effect, which means that all functions in the body benefit at the same time. Ultraviolet light has been proven to lower blood pressure, facilitate cardiac output, increase glycogen (complex sugar) stores in the liver, balance blood sugar, improve the body's resistance to infections (as shown by an increase in the number of lymphocytes and phagocytes), enhance the oxygen-carrying capacity of the blood, and increase the production of sex hormones, along with producing many other health benefits.

Sunbathing may be harmful, however, for those who live on a diet rich in acid-forming, highly processed foods and refined fats/oils or the products that contain them. In addition, alcohol, cigarettes, and other mineral- and vitamin-depleting substances, such as prescription medicines and hallucinogenic drugs, can make the skin vulnerable to ultraviolet radiation. After you have cleared your liver and gallbladder from all gallstones, moderate sun exposure will cause you no harm; in fact, it is essential for good health.

Over 42 percent of Americans suffer from vitamin D deficiency, and 47 percent of pregnant women are severely deficient in this important hormone. Their children tend to have weak bones that break easily, even during their childhood years. Many chronic illnesses are due to vitamin D deficiency, including osteoporosis, cancer, and depression.

You cannot stop a vitamin D deficiency by taking supplements. Sunlight is the only real remedy. To make sufficient amounts of vitamin D, dark-skinned people need to spend at least two to three times longer in the sun than do Caucasians. Their skin absorbs sun rays less efficiently, hence their need for extended sun exposure. Not being exposed to enough sunlight puts African-American men, for example, at a much higher risk of developing cancer of the prostate than white Americans. The use of sunscreens, including sunglasses, multiplies this risk.

During the summer period, it is best to avoid direct sun exposure between 10:00 a.m. and 3:00 p.m., whereas during the winter, spring, and fall seasons, this time period may be most beneficial for the body, especially for those who live at higher latitudes.

For maximum benefits, it is best to take a shower before sunbathing. Contrary to common belief, it is important to *avoid* sunscreens. Sunscreens do not only fail to prevent cancer, but they can actually cause it. Sunscreens "successfully" cancel out the sun's positive effects.[31]

Start your sunlight treatment by exposing your entire body (if possible) to direct sunlight for a few minutes, and then increase your exposure time by a few more minutes each day until you reach 20 to 30 minutes. Alternatively, walking in the sun for an hour has similar benefits. This will give you enough sunlight to produce sufficient amounts of vitamin D and to keep your body and mind healthy (provided that you incorporate the basic aspects of a balanced diet and lifestyle). The body can store enough vitamin D during the sunny days of the year to last you through the winter months.

18. Take Liver Herbs

A number of herbs can further improve the performance of the liver and keep this crucial organ nourished and vital. They can be made into a concoction and are best taken as a tea for 10 days during each change of season or at times of acute illness. Although many herbs will help liver function and assist in maintaining clean blood, the following are among the most prominent ones:

Dandelion root (1 oz.)
Comfrey root (½ oz.) *[1]

---

[31] To learn more about the beneficial effects of sunlight and the harmful effects of sunscreens, see *Timeless Secrets of Health and Rejuvenation.*

Licorice root (1 oz.)
Agrimony (1 oz.)
Wild yam root (1 oz.)
Barberry bark (1 oz.)
Bearsfoot (1 oz.)
Tanners oak bark (1 oz.)
Milk thistle herb (1 oz.)

Note:
*1. Contrary to the opinion of some natural health practitioners, I have never
seen any evidence of comfrey's supposed harmful side effects, only
benefits, especially for the liver.
2. For botanical names see *Product Information* at the end of the book.

For maximum effectiveness, it is best to use all these herbs, in combination, if possible. To do this, mix them together in equal parts (except for comfrey root at half the amount), and add 2 tablespoons of this mixture to 24 ounces of water. Let it sit for 6 hours or overnight; then bring the mixture to a boil, letting it simmer for 5 to 10 minutes before straining. If you forget to prepare this tea the night before, bring the mixture to a boil in the morning, let it simmer as indicated above, and strain it. Drink 2 cups of this "herbal tea" per day on an empty stomach, if possible.

Taken on its own, tea made from the bark of the *red lapacho tree,* also known as Pau d'Arco, Ipe Roxa, and Taheebo, has powerful effects on the liver and the immune system. The Native American herb called chaparral, although tasting very bitter, is also an excellent liver and blood purifier.

19. Apply Daily Oil Therapy

Oil therapy is a simple, yet astoundingly effective, method of cleansing the blood. It is effective for numerous disorders, including blood diseases, lung and liver disorders, tooth and gum diseases, headaches, skin diseases, gastric ulcers, intestinal problems, poor appetite, heart and kidney ailments, encephalitis, nervous conditions, poor memory, female disorders, swollen face, and bags under the eyes. The therapy consists of swishing oil in the mouth.

To apply this therapy you need cold-pressed, unrefined sunflower, sesame, or olive oil. In the morning, preferably after awakening or anytime before breakfast, put 1 tablespoon of oil in your mouth, but do not swallow it. Slowly swish the oil in your mouth, chew it, and draw it through your teeth for 3 to 4 minutes. This thoroughly mixes the oil with saliva and activates the released enzymes. The enzymes draw toxins out of the blood. For this reason, it is important to spit out the oil after no more than 3 to 4 minutes. You do not want any of the released toxins to be reabsorbed. You will find that the oil takes on a milky white or yellowish color as it becomes saturated with toxins and with billions of destructive bacteria.

For best results, repeat this process two more times. Then rinse out your mouth with ½ teaspoon of baking soda, or ½ teaspoon of unrefined sea salt (take either of these dissolved in a small amount of water). This solution will remove all remnants of the oil and toxins. Additionally, you may want to brush your teeth to make sure your mouth is clean. Tongue scraping is also advised.

Some of the visible effects of oil swishing include the elimination of gum bleeding and the whitening of teeth. During times of illness, this procedure can be repeated 3 times per day, but only on an empty stomach. Oil therapy greatly relieves and supports liver functions, as it takes toxins out of the blood that the liver has not been able to remove or detoxify. This benefits the entire organism. If you feel discomfort, only do this once a day.

20. Replace All Metal Tooth Fillings

Metal dentalware is a constant source of poisoning and, possibly, allergic reaction in the body. All metal corrodes in time, especially in the mouth where high concentrations of air and moisture are always present. Mercury amalgam fillings release their extremely toxic compounds and vapor into the body, a reason why German dentists are prohibited by law from giving them to pregnant women. This product has been banned in a number of European countries.

If mercury is considered dangerous for a mother and her baby, it must be considered dangerous for everyone. The liver and kidneys, in particular, which have to deal with noxious substances, such as those released by metal fillings, become gradually poisoned. Cadmium, for example, which is used to make the pink color in dentures, is five times as toxic as lead. It does not take much of it to raise one's blood pressure to abnormal levels. Thallium, which is also found in mercury amalgam fillings, causes leg pain and paraplegia. It affects the skin and the nervous and cardiovascular systems. All wheelchair patients who have been tested for metal poisoning tested positive for thallium. Many people who were in a wheelchair several years after they received metal fillings, completely recovered after all metal was removed from their mouths. Thallium is lethal at a dose of 0.5 to 1.0 gram.

Other elements contained in metal fillings are known for their cancer-producing (carcinogenic) effects. These include nickel, which is used in gold crowns, braces, and children's crowns, and chromium. All metals corrode (including gold, silver, and platinum), and the body absorbs them. Women with breast cancer have often accumulated large amounts of dissolved metals in their breasts. Once the mouth is cleared of all metals, they will also leave the breasts. Likewise, most cysts will shrink and disappear by themselves.

The body's immune system naturally responds to the presence of toxic metals in the body and, eventually, develops allergic reactions. These allergies may show up as a sinus condition, tinnitus, enlarged neck and glands, bloating, enlarged spleen, arthritic conditions, headaches and migraines, eye diseases, and even more serious complications, such as paralysis or heart attacks. An obvious way to improve all these conditions is to replace all metal fillings with composite fillings that contain *no* metals.[32] If you need major dental work, such as a crown, root canal, bridge, or implant, it is best to seek an alternative dentist who uses the least-harmful dental procedures available. Additionally, cleanse the liver and kidneys, and drink tea made from liver herbs (see above recipe) for 10 days after replacing a filling.

---

[32] For details on composite fillings, see *Timeless Secrets of Health and Rejuvenation* by the author.

21. Bring Balance to Your Emotional Health

On a deeper level, every physically manifested ailment *is* an imbalanced emotion. Emotions are signals of comfort or discomfort that our body sends us at every moment of our conscious existence. They contain specific vibrations that serve as a kind of weather report, telling us how we feel about ourselves, about others, and about what is "good" or "bad," "right" or "wrong," both in our lives and in our world. Emotions are like reflections from a mirror that reveal to us everything we need to know to go through the trials and tribulations of life. Our body, which can only be *felt,* is precisely such an emotional mirror or messenger. A dirty mirror reflects only certain parts of us or makes us look distorted. If we are emotionally stuck and unable to understand what is happening to us, it is because we are not open to listen to, understand, and follow the messages that our body is trying to convey to us.

All emotional problems indicate a lack of awareness. If we are not completely aware why these emotions and/or physical challenges are there, we are out of touch with ourselves and, hence, are incapable of making positive changes in our life. Many people are so disconnected from their feelings that they do not even know *what* they feel. Practicing mindfulness brings our attention back to where we are and who we are. By staying *with* our emotions for as long as they last, we can unleash the tremendous creative powers that lie dormant within us. Emotions are not there to be judged or suppressed; they are there to be understood and accepted. As we learn to observe them, we will begin to understand their true meaning. Instead of unconsciously *reacting* to a difficult situation or person, we will be able to *act* consciously out of our own free will.

Emotions want to be acknowledged because they are the only way our body can tell us how we truly feel about others and ourselves. By accepting and honoring all our feelings and emotions, rather than repressing them, we begin to experience a different reality in life, one that offers us freedom from judgment and freedom from pain. We will begin to see a sense and purpose in everything that is happening to us, regardless of whether it is "right" or "wrong," "good" or "bad." This eliminates fear, as well as all the other emotions that arise from fear. Balancing our emotions is one of the most important nonphysical ways we have to attain a sound state of health, happiness, and peacefulness.

The approaches, messages, and artwork contained in my book *Lifting the Veil of Duality* have been designed to bring balance to your emotional health. (See *Other Books, Products, and Services by the Author.*) In fact, your entire perception of problems, limitations, disease, pain, and suffering may become profoundly altered after reading that book. In addition, what formerly may have led you to age faster, or perhaps even experience a physical illness, may rapidly become transmuted into powerful opportunities to generate joy, abundance, vitality, and rejuvenation throughout the rest of your life. My healing system, Sacred Santémony, described at the end of the book, is a highly effective method to balance the root causes of emotional imbalances.

In the meantime, you may greatly benefit from following this simple procedure for balancing emotions: Transfer your mind back to a beautiful period in your early childhood, perhaps when you were three years old. Remember how very free and joyful you were. You had no preconceived notions of what was right or wrong, good or bad, beautiful or ugly. See yourself interacting with other people with wonder, total ease, and innocent openness. You are interested in all there is, and you feel safe, nourished, and loved. Now go forward in time to a situation in your life where you no longer felt this way, where you felt a lack of love or were ignored, rebuked, criticized, or abused. Notice the contraction and coldness in your heart. Once again, go back to the innocent spirit of your childlike nature and bring it into that situation that caused you so much pain. Fill yourself with that three-year- old innocence and untainted joy, and radiate it all around you. See it filling everyone with that same joyful radiance. Now move to another event in your life that caused you unhappiness, and repeat this process. Go through every difficulty or negative experience in your life, and heal it with your three-year-old joyful self.

This exercise is so effective because, in reality, there is no linear time. Time is merely a concept we use to separate events that have already happened, are occurring right now, or may unfold sometime in the future. Thus, in truth, past events have just as powerful an effect on us today as they had then. For this reason, there is so much fear, tension, stress, anger, conflict, and violence in our world. Most people cannot let go of their past experiences and, therefore, re-create similar scenarios to deal with them in one way or another. However, by undoing their negative impact through this simple exercise of self-empowerment, you can literally change your past and, thereby, your present and future realities.

It may take one to two weeks (20 to 30 minutes per day) to sift through and heal all your past unbalanced emotions in this way, but it is worthwhile. Whenever you react negatively to something in your life, it is because you have had an unbalanced emotional experience before that. By balancing all the unwanted experiences that have occurred between your early childhood and this moment, you can help remove many of the root causes of any existing emotional, mental, physical, and spiritual problems and can prevent new ones from arising.

Chapter 6

What Can I Expect from the Liver and Gallbladder Flush?

A Disease-Free Life

Disease is not part of the body's design. Symptoms of disease merely indicate that the body is trying to prevent serious harm or even a life-threatening situation from occurring. We become sick when our immune system is suppressed and overburdened with accumulated toxic waste. The response of the body to this type of extreme congestion is to clear the toxins in a number of different, and usually unpleasant, ways. The body's methods of self-defense and cleansing often require pain, fever, infection, inflammation, and ulceration. In more serious cases, cancer and a buildup of plaque inside the arterial walls help avert the ill person's imminent demise.[33] Most types of internal "suffocation" are preceded or accompanied by a blockage of the liver bile ducts. When the liver, which is the main factory and detoxification center of the body, becomes congested with gallstones, disease is a likely outcome.

When you clear the liver bile ducts from all obstructions and then adopt and maintain a balanced diet and lifestyle, your body naturally returns to a state of balance (homeostasis). This balanced state is what most people call "good health." The old saying "An ounce of prevention is worth a pound of cure" applies most appropriately to the liver. If the liver is kept free of gallstones, the body's balanced state is unlikely to be upset. Having a clean liver means having a clean bill of health.

---

[33] To learn more about the four major causes of disease, how disease develops, and the true reasons for cancer, heart disease, diabetes, and AIDS, refer to *Timeless Secrets of Health and Rejuvenation.*

Health insurance companies and their clients could greatly benefit from the liver and gallbladder flush in several important ways. These companies would be able to lower their premium rates and expenditures considerably, while the insured population would enjoy much better health, fewer sick days from work, and freedom from the fear and pain that typically accompany disease. Older generations would no longer be considered a burden, as they would be able to take care of themselves more and more rather than less and less. Health care costs could be cut drastically, which may be the only way to safeguard continued progress and prosperity in nations such as the United States and the United Kingdom. If the current trend of escalating health expenditures in the United States continues to grow as fast as it has in recent decades, major corporations are likely to end up bankrupt if they continue to offer health insurance as a benefit to their employees. In 2001, the cost of health care in the United States exceeded the $1 trillion mark, and in 2004, total health care spending amounted to $1.9 trillion. That represented 16 percent of the nation's GDP, and there is no end to this trend in sight. Healthcare spending is projected to double to $4 trillion over the next decade.

Good health care cannot be measured by how much money is being spent on treating symptoms of disease. Treating the symptoms of an illness inevitably requires further treatments, because the origins of disease are ignored and become worse if left unattended. According to the premise of modern medicine, to "successfully" treat symptoms, which implies suppressing the body's own healing efforts, a patient needs to take recourse to poisonous drugs, radiation, or surgery. All these forms of medical intervention have harmful side effects, which in turn become the cause of new diseases that require further treatment. The quick-fix approach of suppressing symptoms of disease is a major cause of chronic illness, premature death, and, of course, spiraling health care costs. Over 900,000 people die each year unnecessarily as a direct result of side-effects from expensive medical treatments. By comparison, it is very inexpensive to actually cure disease and prevent new diseases from arising. Conventional health care is becoming less and less affordable for most people in the world and is likely to become a rare privilege for a relative few in the future. If the liver and gallbladder flush were being prescribed by doctors in the United States, even just to patients with gallbladder disease, it could help each of the 20 million gallstone sufferers to live a normal, comfortable life and eliminate or prevent numerous other related illnesses.

The liver flush does much more than merely restore proper gallbladder and liver functions; it helps people take active care of their health for the rest of their lives. Taking out an insurance policy against disease cannot guarantee a disease-free life. Good health develops naturally when you keep the body free of gallstones and other toxic waste deposits, and when you fulfill the most basic requirements for maintaining youthfulness and vitality throughout life.

Improved Digestion, Energy, and Vitality

"Good digestion" comprises three basic processes in the body:

- Ingested food is broken down into its nutrient components.
- Nutrients are absorbed and distributed to all the cells and then metabolized efficiently.
- The waste products resulting from the breakdown and utilization of food are all eliminated through the excretory organs and systems.

The body requires good digestion in order to guarantee continuous, efficient turnover of its 60 to 100 trillion cells. To sustain homeostasis, the body needs to make 30 billion new cells each day to replace the same number of old, worn-out, or damaged cells. If this process occurs smoothly, day after day and year after year, the new generations of cells in the body will be as effective and healthy as the previous ones. Even if certain cells, such as brain and heart cells, cannot be replaced (this theory is about to become obsolete), their constituents, such as carbon, oxygen, hydrogen, and nitrogen atoms (all of which make up the air we breathe), are nevertheless renewed continuously.

The natural turnover of cells or atoms, however, is no longer complete or efficient in the majority of people who live in a fast-paced world that has little time for a healthy lifestyle and balanced diet. People are unhealthy today because they eat unhealthy foods (and think unhealthy thoughts). In contrast, a nourishing diet consists of natural, unpolluted foods and fresh, clean water. Only very few societies have managed to maintain their youth and health at all age levels. Such peoples live in remote and secluded areas, such as the Abkhasian Mountains in Southern Russia; the Himalayan Mountains in India, Tibet, and China; the Andes in South America; and in parts of northern Mexico.. Their diet consists only of pure, fresh foods. Thankfully, you don't need to live in remote areas of the world to be healthy. In fact, it is very normal, for example, to have completely clean blood vessels at age 100 or older (see **Figure 14**).

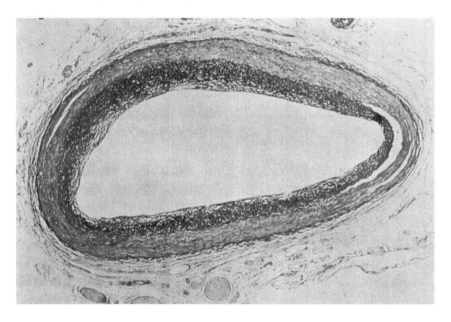

Figure 14: Open artery of a 100-year-old American woman

By cleansing our body and giving it the best possible treatment, we can all raise our quality of life to a high level of energy and vitality, which is the natural state of health that every human being deserves. A well-functioning digestive system and gallstone-free liver provide the main conditions through which the body can regulate the smooth turnover of cells without accumulating toxins. This is the best antidote to aging and disease any person can have.

Freedom from Pain

Pain is a signal that the body uses to identify and correct certain problems or malfunctioning in the organs, systems, muscles, and joints. Pain is not a disease in itself, but instead is the sign of a proper immune response to an abnormal situation. An abnormal situation could mean congestion of lymph, blood, and waste matter. Any physical congestion leads to a poor supply of oxygen. Oxygen-deprived tissues almost always signal pain. When the pain subsides naturally through cleansing or the body's removing the congestion (without the use of painkillers), it shows that the body has returned to a state of balance. Chronic pain indicates that the immune response and self-cleansing ability of the body is not sufficient and that the cause of the problem is still active and intact.

Cleansing the liver and gallbladder of all gallstones can help to reduce and eliminate pain in the body, regardless of whether it is located in the joints, head, nerves, muscles, or organs. The body is only as healthy as the blood and lymph are. If the blood and lymph contain large amounts of toxins, as occurs when there is congestion in the liver, then irritation, inflammation and infection, or damage to cells and tissues in the weakest parts of body may result. If the functions of digestion, metabolism, and the elimination of waste materials in the body are impaired as a result of poor liver performance, the *immune system* cannot accomplish its healing work in the body.

The healing response is dependent on the efficiency of the immune system, the greatest part of which is located in the intestinal tract. The liver, which is the main organ controlling digestion and cellular metabolism, must be free of all obstructions (gallstones) in order to prevent the immune system from being stressed and overtaxed. If immunity is low in the intestines, it will also be depressed in all other parts of the body. Pain relief occurs automatically once congestion subsides and the immune system returns to its full power and efficiency. Pain is not something that requires treatment, unless it is unbearable. You would not try fighting the darkness of the night when all you need to do is to switch on the light. It is, in fact, unwise to kill the messenger (pain) that tries to warn you about an approaching enemy. Since chronic pain is caused by chronic congestion, the liver, intestines, kidneys, and lymphatic system should be cleansed before attempting to treat the pain. In almost every case, this approach relieves all pain and restores vibrant health along with proper immune functions.

A More Flexible Body

Physical flexibility is a measure of how well the organs, joints, muscles, connective tissues, and cells are nourished by the food we eat, the water we drink, and the air we breathe. The digestive and metabolic processes that make these nutrients and substances available to the cells need to be in top condition for health to be a real and long-lasting outcome. Stiffness in the joints and muscles indicates the presence of acidic metabolic waste products in these parts of the body owing to poor digestive and eliminative functions.

Anyone who practices yoga, gymnastics, or any other form of exercise and does several liver flushes will notice greatly increased flexibility of the spine, joints, and muscles. Deposits of mineral salts in the neck and shoulder areas begin to lessen, and aches and stiffness disappear. The whole body feels more "connected," as the connective tissues that keep the cells together become more supple and fluid again.

A river of pure, clean water flows more easily and with less friction than a river that is filled with filth and mud. One of the liver's most important functions is to keep the blood thin so that it can distribute nutrients to the cells, collect waste materials, and carry messenger hormones to their destinations on time. Thick blood is a common denominator for most illnesses in the body, and you can recognize it by a lack of flexibility in certain parts of the body, along with other symptoms, including tiredness. If the spine and joints are permanently stiff and painful, this indicates that most of the internal organs are suffering from circulatory problems. Blood circulation greatly improves when gallstones cease to congest the liver. This leads to increased flexibility and mobility throughout the body. A good and regular exercise program helps to support and maintain this newly found flexibility.

A flexible body also suggests that the mind is open and adaptable. A rigid body, by contrast, is a sign of a rigid and fearful mind. As the body is supplied with thinner blood, and as hardened structures begin to soften again, your mental attitude also becomes more expansive and accommodating. This enhances your ability to flow with the opportunities of life in the present moment, adding greater joy and fulfillment to each new day.

Reversal of the Aging Process

Many people view aging as an unavoidable phenomenon that, like a disease, will afflict them eventually. However, this viewpoint applies only to its "negative" consequences. You can just as well see aging as a positive growth process that makes life richer, increases wisdom, and enhances experience and maturity—all assets that are rarely found in one's youth. The negative aspect of the aging process, with which the majority of people identify, is a metabolic disorder that develops gradually over a period of time.

The unwanted effects of aging result from malfunctioning that occurs on the cellular level. When the body's cells are unable to remove their daily-generated metabolic waste material fast enough, some of it is deposited in the cell membranes. In fact, the cell membranes become cellular "garbage cans." The cells cannot rid themselves of all their own waste because the surrounding connective tissue is congested with other waste material (owing to lymphatic blockage). In due time, inefficient waste disposal becomes more pronounced and apparent in the body. The withheld waste gradually cuts off the cells' supply of oxygen, nutrients, and water, and increasingly thickens their membranes. The cell membranes of a newborn baby are very thin, nearly colorless, and transparent. The average 70-year-old person today has cell membranes that are at least five times as thick as are those found in a baby's body. The membranes' color is generally brown and, in some cases, even black. This cell-degenerative process is what we generally refer to as "aging."

During normal aging, which begins right from the beginning of life, all cells in the body are routinely replaced with new cells. On the other hand, during abnormal aging, the newly created cells are not as healthy as the old ones were. The affected tissues or groups of cells have become weaker and suffer malnutrition, thereby giving the new generation of cells a poor start in life. Consequently, before long, the membranes of the new cells also become clogged up. They have no chance to develop into healthy young cells. As more and more of the cells and the surrounding connective tissues become saturated with toxic substances, entire organs in the body begin to age and deteriorate as well.

The skin, which is the largest organ in the body, also begins to suffer from malnourishment. Consequently, it may lose some of its former elasticity, change its natural color, become dry and rough, and develop blemishes that consist of metabolic waste products. At this stage, the negative aspect of the aging process becomes visible on the outside. Therefore, it is obvious that external aging, which is a direct result of defective cell metabolism, starts inside the body.

Impaired digestion and liver function are the main causes of inefficient cell metabolism. Both functions improve dramatically when *all* existing gallstones in the liver and gallbladder are eliminated and other toxic waste materials are removed from the organs, tissues, and cells through simple methods of cleansing (as discussed in this book). As soon as the cells begin to shed their "dark skin" (a natural result of the cleansing), the absorption of oxygen, nutrients, and water increases, and so does cell vitality. As digestion and metabolism continue to improve, instead of being old and tired, the cells will become young and dynamic again. This is the time when the aging process actually reverses, and the positive aspects of aging begin to dominate.

Inner and Outer Beauty

The results of steadily improving cell metabolism will affect the way you feel about your inner self as much as they will show on the outside. Older people look radiant and youthful when they are truly healthy. Young people can look quite old if their bodies are toxic and tired. Naturally, if you want to achieve outer beauty, you must develop inner beauty first.

If your body has accumulated a lot of waste material, it is not capable of imbuing you with a sense of beauty and worthiness. There are still groups of indigenous people living in the most remote parts of the world who enjoy perfect health and vitality. They regularly purge their liver, kidneys, and intestines with oils, herbs, and fluids. These practices have become lost to modern societies whose main emphasis is on improving the superficial physical appearance and, in the case of an illness, fixing its symptoms rather than removing its cause.

Those who have done a series of liver flushes report that they feel much better about their body, their life, and their environment. In many cases, the person's self-esteem and ability to appreciate others improves as the body becomes increasingly purified. The liver flush can greatly contribute toward developing vitality and inner beauty. This will not only help to slow or reverse the aging process, but will also make you feel more youthful and attractive, regardless of your age.

Improved Emotional Health

The liver flush has direct implications on how you feel about yourself and others. Under stress, you are likely to become irritable, annoyed, frustrated, and even angry. Most people assume that stress has something to do with the external problems they face in their lives. Yet this is only partially true. Our response to certain issues, situations, or people is only negative because we are not able to cope with them.

The liver, which maintains the nervous system by supplying it with vital nutrients, also determines our stress response. Gallstones impede the proper distribution of nutrients, which forces the body to take recourse to several emergency measures, including the excessive secretion of stress hormones. For a short while, this quick first-aid measure helps to maintain most bodily functions, but eventually the body's equilibrium becomes disturbed and the nervous system is thrown off balance. Given this imbalanced state of affairs, any external pressure or demanding situation may trigger an exaggerated stress response that, in turn, may give rise to the feeling of being stressed or overwhelmed.

Our emotional health is intimately linked to our physical health. Cleansing the liver and keeping it clean helps maintain emotional balance. When you remove your gallstones you also root out any deep-seated anger and resentment that may have been stored there for a long time (the body holds onto various emotions in different body parts). The relief that comes with letting go of past, unresolved issues may create a new sense of being alive. Moreover, the feelings of freedom and euphoria that you commonly experience almost immediately after a liver flush, indicate what can lie in store for you once your liver and gallbladder are completely cleansed.

A Clearer Mind and Improved Creativity

Clarity of mind, memory recall, creativity, and the ability to concentrate and focus attention all depend on how well the brain and nervous system are nourished. An ineffective circulatory system has a dulling and suppressing effect on all mental processes. This, in turn, stresses and strains the nervous system.

With each new liver flush you undertake, you are likely to notice a further improvement in your mental faculties. Many people report that their mind becomes less turbulent and more relaxed. Others report a sudden influx of expansive thoughts that help to improve their work performance and creative output. Artists generally find an opening of a new dimension to their creative expression, including a more acute perception of colors, shapes, and forms.

Those involved in techniques of spiritual growth or self-improvement will find that the elimination of all gallstones in the liver may help them to gain access to deeper, formerly hidden areas within themselves and to use more of their mental potential. The liver flush particularly helps balance the *solar plexus chakra.* The solar plexus represents the energy center in the body responsible for willpower, energy absorption, and distribution, as well as functions of the liver, gallbladder, stomach, pancreas, and spleen. This central switchboard for physical and emotional activities becomes far more comfortable after doing a series of liver flushes.

Chapter 7

What People Say About the Liver Flush

"The liver flush, what a difference it makes! I'm a 46-year-old woman and have had health problems practically all my life. As a child, my health problems were minor, but numerous and constant. It was not until I became an adult that my minor problems became major ones. My road to good health has been long and exceptionally difficult. I have been probed with cameras, pricked with needles, scanned, x-rayed, and injected with dyes, and have undergone five operations. I have been prescribed and consumed vast amounts of medications of various dosages, ranging from high to exceptionally high, especially antibiotics. I would always get better for a while, but my problems continued, each time reappearing in different areas of my body with worse symptoms than before.

"Finally, after exhausting myself with the whole medical system and absolutely at my wit's end, I decided to consider natural health. I read everything I could get my hands on, stopped my prescribed medication, changed my diet, and underwent a series of colonics. It began to work, my health improved dramatically, but still I needed more. I did not have any energy and my diet had to be strictly adhered to in order to prevent my digestion problems from returning. Then one day, a friend, God bless her, gave me a book she thought I might be interested in reading, *The Amazing Liver and Gallbladder Flush*! At present I have completed six flushes. It's not quite complete, but the difference is so noticeable that I can speak about it with great confidence. The last six months have been truly amazing for me.

"So far I have passed about 2,000 stones ranging from the size of a pea to a golf ball. In addition, I gained extra, unexpected benefits by passing a small tumor and various types of parasites. My change from being fragile and sickly, to vibrant and strong, is astounding. My digestion has completely changed to that of a normal functioning individual, something I've never experienced before. I have suffered from sinus problems as long as I can remember; now they are gradually normalizing, as my allergies disappear. My friends and family have all witnessed the dramatic changes in me, and can't believe the abundant energy I have. Both my physical and mental changes are so extraordinary; I just want to announce it to the world. Life just doesn't get any better than that! On a daily basis, I am thankful and compelled to share *The Amazing Liver and Gallbladder Flush* with anyone wanting natural self-help and a new life. These feelings I have are still so new to me, I wake up every morning thinking it was just a dream. My dream has come true! Life without health is no life at all. It's truly remarkable and my life has finally begun!!"

Debbie Perez, Germany

"I completed my tenth liver flush about three weeks ago, and this last one was clear of any stones. I have removed in excess of 9,000 stones over a period of about twelve months. My health is so much better; no tiredness, boundless energy. For the twelve months prior to starting the cleanse, I had suffered one illness after another, countless *Whitlow* infections of the fingers which saw me hospitalized for I.V. antibodies. Then I developed chickenpox, followed by shingles which have left me with some battle scarring. Soon *Encephalitis* followed which affected my vision. I have to say that at that stage my will to recover was not very strong. My bowel movements were loose for some time. I also developed a nasty infection of the mouth which, according to my dentist, has eaten away at my jawbone. But now I am back to feeling pretty damn good and it's thanks to you and your wonderful book. With my very best wishes."

Robert M., UK

"A client of mine, age 33, is a nice man who had a benign brain tumor removed two years ago and [suffered from] headaches since the age of 10. A year after the operation the pain was still a big problem; he would miss work for days, and end up cold, shivering and sweaty in bed. His original surgeon opened his head again a year ago to 'relieve fluid pressure' (as a CST, I can do that with my hands!). The headaches persisted and he would have his 'funny heads' where he would experience waves of tingling for 30 seconds a few times every day, quite a problem while driving. So I suggested some liver flushes of which he has now done two. The three weeks since the last flush have been 'the best for many years,' no headaches or 'funny heads,' his complexion is clear and healthy, eyes bright and clear, he feels great. The number of stones passed was many thousands in the second flush; he could not believe what came out. He's really grateful and delighted with the results and the book."

Geoffrey M., Health Practitioner, UK

"Just thought you would like to hear the latest report from my cardiologist, whom I went to see on Monday, just because it has now been over one year since my heart attack." This was the beginning of an e-mail message that Susan, a 62-year-old client of mine from Arizona, sent me recently. "He was a bit disturbed when I first saw him," she continued, "because I said I was not taking any medications and had not since last August. As he was talking with me he said he would probably prescribe a couple of medications for me to start taking again, but first he wanted to do an echocardiogram and a stress test.

"I agreed to them both and they were done in his office. While I was on the treadmill, I became tired, so I told his assistants I was getting tired and they said, 'You may be, but your heart is not!' They said the echocardiogram and stress test were well within normal limits. When the cardiologist came back in the room he said, 'I am totally surprised, just totally surprised. These tests show a healthy heart, no damage at all! So you can go home, continue doing what you have been doing and come back to see me in six months.' He did not mention anything else about medications."

Her message ended by saying how grateful she was for having received all the advice and recommendations that had given her the power to claim a healthy normal heart. Susan is one of thousands of people who were listed as incurable heart disease patients, but through liver flushing and changes in diet and lifestyle have beaten the odds.

Susan M., Arizona

"I have had gallstones for approximately 15 years. The first time I did the flush, I got out literally thousands of stones. The last ones came out all clumped together about the size of my fist. It was absolutely painless."

P. B., Spain

"I am a 46-year-old manager of a Midwestern development company who requires medication for hyperthyroidism. As a result, I need to have my blood value tested twice yearly to monitor my endocrine system. Two years ago, blood tests also showed elevated cholesterol level of 229 mg% [200 mg per 100 ml]. My endocrinologist wanted to put me on a cholesterol-lowering drug called Lipitor,[34] which I steadfastly refused.

"I subsequently visited with Andreas Moritz where I learnt to adjust my diet and cleanse my liver. After completing two liver flushes my blood cholesterol levels dropped to 177 mg%. My 65-year-old doctor couldn't believe the result. He has never seen such a rapid turnaround. He was intrigued and wanted to learn more about the liver flush.

"In addition, my required dosage of Synthyroid® for my hypothyroidism has been reduced from 0.175 to 0.125 mg during the past two years, with further reductions coming. I recently finished my sixth liver flush and I look forward to continued improvements of my health and vitality."

Bryant Wangard, Minnesota

"The day after my colonic, after passing about 150 gallstones, I felt something surge into my colon all at once. I then felt this mass slowly moving from the beginning to the end of my colon, a very strange feeling. Anyway, it got to the end but wouldn't come out. I

---

[34] For more information on Lipitor and high cholesterol, see Chapter 1.

waited two days and when nothing happened I took colosan.[35] The third day I had a bowel movement, mostly pulverized by colosan, but after washing the dark sludge away there was a huge gallstone inside. It was the size of a golf ball, along with several others the size of a quarter. I couldn't believe it. I called my therapist and requested another colonic, as I didn't feel I was finished. I got the colonic and to my surprise I passed about another 100 dime-size stones. I thought for sure this was it; but during the past four days I've passed a few more stones with each bowel movement. I think when it ended I must have passed around 1,000 stones all together, large, medium and tiny. Whew, what a trip, I just don't see how so many stones so large could be inside such a small body. My energy level has dramatically increased and my abdomen area is so flat and soft. I feel like a million bucks."

D. P., Germany

"I have recently completed my ninth liver flush and am extremely excited about the results. Towards the evening of the day of that flush I passed a calcified gallstone that measured a little less than 2½ inches in length and 1½ inches in width (see **Figure 6b**), followed by about 100 smaller, but equally calcified gallstones. Apparently, these gallstones had totally filled up my gallbladder for many years and, thereby, prevented my liver from properly detoxifying my blood and body. After each successive flush I have eliminated hundreds of stones and the immediate impact has been tremendous: whiter, shiny eyes; a happier disposition; markedly reduced levels of frustration and anger; and improved digestive capability. But nothing had prepared me for what my ninth flush did for me. The aches and pains I used to have throughout my body for so many years left me overnight, including the chronic stiffness in my neck/shoulder, back and joints. When lightly pressed upon during a massage, Shiatsu session or chiropractic adjustment, almost every part of my body used to respond with strong pain. Now there is no more pain, whatsoever.

---

[35] Colosan is an effective colon cleanser, described in *Timeless Secrets of Health and Rejuvenation*.

"Before I started this cleansing regime, I was on over a dozen different medical drugs and vitamin supplements. After only one liver flush I was able to stop taking my thyroid medication which I had been on for five years.

"As a middle-aged baby boomer entering menopause, I have been surprised to have my menstrual cycle return immediately after a few of the flushes, suggesting that the premature onset of menopause, in my case, may have been accelerated because of a congested liver and colon. Other startlingly wonderful benefits have been an increased sex drive and feelings of sexiness, decreased desire for junk foods and overall youthful attitude—far more joyful and optimistic than I've felt in 10 years. My deep gratitude goes to Andreas Moritz for bringing this invaluable aide to our attention and, in this instance, saving my life!"

L. M., California

"Until flush #11, I really didn't have much to say except I released over 2,000 stones. However, since the last flush, my face has been completely clear of acne for more than 13 days (and counting!) for the first time since I was 14 years old. This is a major physical breakthrough for me because for 22 years I have dreaded looking in the mirror each morning. Although in my adult years the acne has been relatively mild, it was still a nuisance. High school was painful because of the major breakouts. I consider it a miracle that I can look someone in the eyes and not be self-conscious of my face. It is a terrific feeling!"

P. V., Minnesota

"I've done the liver flush four times so far and gotten a lot of stones out. I was advised to have urgent surgery last October, but my pain has gone away and my digestion keeps getting better."

Alexi, USA

My Story:

"When I was eight years old, my uncle—who was the leading iridologist[36] in Germany at that time—examined my eyes and told me that I had 'stones' in my liver. From age 6, I began to have difficulties digesting food. During the following twelve years, I developed such varied problems as juvenile rheumatoid arthritis, arrhythmia, chronic constipation, chronic headaches and migraines, frightening nightmares, anemia, skin diseases, and a short scoliosis of the spine. Every four to five weeks, I suffered fainting spells during mass at church or while waiting in line at a bank or post office. These fainting spells became more and more severe and were accompanied by vomiting and diarrhea. I was sick in bed for three to four days following each of these episodes. No doctor was able to offer an explanation for these debilitating symptoms.

"At age 15, I began to seriously study the digestive system, and I changed my diet numerous times in order to find out whether my choice of foods contributed in some way to my ailments. Eventually, I realized that I had literally been poisoning my body with foods derived from animal sources (meat, fish, chicken, eggs, cheese, and milk). After I completely avoided these foods, most of my symptoms disappeared, including the arthritis and arrhythmia. However, my liver seemed sluggish, the scoliosis remained, and I was heading toward another series of crises. About ten years later my fainting spells progressed into major gallbladder attacks. The stones that my uncle had seen years earlier had grown larger and increased in number. [*Note:* If the stones are not completely removed, they continue to block bile flow, which increases stone formation.] In total, I suffered over forty extremely painful attacks that lasted three to ten days each. These were usually accompanied by vomiting and diarrhea, headaches, excruciating backaches, and sleepless nights. Since I had never taken painkillers, medical drugs, or vaccines in my life, they were not an option for me. Besides, I was determined to discover a true solution to this problem.

---

[36] Iridology, or the science of eye interpretation, is a medically accepted, diagnostic method in Germany and several other countries. It can quickly reveal the existence and causes of physical ailments through careful study of the iris.

"I began to experiment with different herbs, treatments, and liver-cleansing methods prevalent in various cultures around the world for thousands of years. From all the methods I researched, tested, tried, and improved upon, the procedure outlined in this book turned out to be the most effective for me. During my first real liver flush, I passed over 500 gallstones. My gallbladder attacks ended that very day. Other problems, such as backaches, joint pain, short scoliosis, and digestive problems, improved with each new flush. After twelve flushes and passing 3,500 gallstones, my liver was completely clean and, at last, my health was the way I had always wanted it to be. Today people comment on my youthful vitality, zest for life, and fit, flexible body, things I only dreamed about having thirtyfive years ago."

Chapter 8

Frequently Asked Questions

The following are some of the most frequently asked questions with corresponding answers regarding gallstones, the liver and gallbladder flush, and colon health.

Q. Could it be that it is natural or even advantageous to have a certain amount of gallstones in the liver?

A. Certainly not. Bile ducts transport bile from the liver cells toward the intestinal tract, similar to water pipes delivering water to a home or field. To block the bile ducts with gallstones cuts off oxygen and the supply of nutrients to the liver cells. This goes against the very design of the body. Therefore, there is no advantage to having the bile ducts clogged up. Bile also carries toxins out of the liver; congested bile ducts obstruct this vital function, damaging the liver and leading to overall toxicity in the body. The only "purpose" of gallstones in the liver is to trap and neutralize poisons that otherwise could enter and damage the intestines. However, as I have repeatedly shown in earlier chapters, this impedes the liver's function, leading to detrimental effects throughout the body.

Q. I passed stones several days after the colonic following my last liver flush and felt very tired until they were all gone. How can I ensure that the stones that come out of the liver also leave my body?

A. Most people eliminate any remaining stones during the post–liver-flush colonic. If you continue to feel dullness in the head, tiredness, or other symptoms of toxicity in the body, use one of the intestinal cleansers such as colosan, aloe vera juice, castor oil, and the like. Discontinue their use once the discomfort subsides. In some cases of intestinal strictures or other major congestion, a second colonic may be necessary. These difficulties, albeit rare, usually occur due to a "spastic colon," a chronic condition in a segment of the large intestine that inhibits bowel movements.

Q. I am pregnant. Is it okay for me to do the liver flush?

A. Although the liver flush has no known side effects on mother and baby, to be on the safe side, it is better to postpone the flush until at least six weeks after delivery. For future pregnancies, however, I recommend that before you conceive, you eliminate all gallstones through a series of liver flushes. This will ensure optimal health for both yourself and your baby during and after the pregnancy. Having said this, I know of several pregnant women who have done successful liver flushes without a problem.

Q. I cannot tolerate apple juice. Is there an alternative?

A. The malic acid in apple juice seems to have the best properties for preparing the liver and gallbladder to expel gallstones easily and effectively. Try to drink the apple juice very slowly and/or water it down. If you still cannot tolerate apple juice, you may substitute 1,500 to 2,000 mg of malic acid powder dissolved in two glasses of water. Cranberry juice, the herb gold coin grass, and apple cider vinegar are other good alternatives. (See details in Chapter 4.)

Q. Would it be better to do the liver flushes in intervals of two to three weeks or spread them over a longer period of time, say one every two or three months?

A. This is up to you to decide. I recommend that, once you have started liver flushing, you continue cleansing at regular intervals until all gallstones are removed. Sometimes, not cleansing for two months or more can make the next flush more difficult and less successful. After a liver flush, it takes about two weeks before enough gallstones have moved from the rear of the liver toward the two hepatic ducts (exiting the liver) to make another purge worthwhile. You may want to do the flush about every three weeks until no more stones come out, or else take a little more time between each flush. If you decide to do a liver flush every two weeks, start drinking the apple juice two weeks after the last main purge. Most people prefer to flush about once per month. In any case, it is important that you get rid of *all* the stones, big and small. Just a few small ones clustered together in one of the larger bile ducts can produce major symptoms of discomfort in the body, such as indigestion, bloating, headaches, backaches, and so on.

Q. Should I avoid doing liver flushes while I am menstruating?

A. Although the liver flush may still be somewhat effective when done during menstruation, it is more convenient and comfortable for women to flush their liver before or after the monthly cycle. Besides, menstrual bleeding is another form of cleansing the body, and it is best for the body not to cleanse on two fronts at the same time.

Q. Is it really necessary to have a colonic irrigation before and after each liver flush?

A. For optimum results, the liver flush should always be preceded and followed by some form of colonic cleansing. (See also *Keep Your Colon Clean* in Chapter 5.) The quickest and most reliable method of freeing the colon of spastic or congested areas is colonic irrigation. Once the colonic therapist tells you that your colon is clean, you can skip the colonic prior to liver flushing and replace it with one of the other methods of colon cleansing. However, continue having colonics after each liver flush, ideally within three days. The postcolonic eliminates any gallstones that may have been trapped in the colon. Experience shows that there are always some stones left behind, which could become a source of toxicity, irritation, or inflammation. I strongly recommend that you do not do liver flushes without having a colonic or colema afterward.

Q. I have had three liver flushes so far and eliminated a total of about 900 to 1,000 stones of all sizes and colors. Most stones came out during the second and third flushes. When is my liver going to improve?

A. Your liver functions started improving the moment the first stones were expelled. Gallstones congesting the liver bile ducts have a suffocating effect on surrounding liver cells. Releasing the stones through the liver flush helps them "breathe" again, produce more bile, and detoxify the blood more efficiently. Although the larger bile ducts keep blocking up again as the smaller bile ducts pass their stones into them, eventually they will also be cleared (through repeated cleansing). Once all stones are removed, the liver as a whole can repair itself and restore normal functions. This is when you will notice lasting benefits.

Q. How long does it take to receive the full benefits from completing a series of, let's say, eight liver flushes?

A. Once your liver has released the last gallstones, your digestive functions will improve significantly, which will benefit every part of your body. This also gives the rest of the body the opportunity to cleanse itself and repair the damage that has occurred due to the accumulation of gallstones in the liver and gallbladder. Any cleansing reactions that may result from the removal of the stones should be regarded as positive side effects. If other causes of ill health have been eliminated as well (see *Simple Guidelines to Avoid Gallstones,* Chapter 5), this phase will be short-lived and replaced by a new sense of well-being and vitality. Once the liver is clean, it takes about six months before all liver functions have returned to normal. Having a clean liver is one of the best guarantees for a disease-free life.

Q. I am 76 years old and suffer from osteoporosis, digestive trouble, and several other ailments. Can someone my age still benefit from the liver flush?

A. Age is no impediment for the body to be healthy. As long as you are breathing, the liver flush can help improve liver functions and, thereby, increase the nutrient and energy supply to the cells of your body. The negative aspect of aging is simply a progressive state of malnourishment and toxicity, both of which can be helped through a series of liver flushes and adjustments to diet. The elderly respond very well to the liver flush and show increased signs of energy, physical mobility, clarity of mind, appetite, sensory enjoyment, and a better sense of self. Apart from improving their physical and mental condition, they often report that they are *"coming to life again."* No elderly person should have to die from a debilitating disease. If the liver flush were to be introduced into retirement homes and care facilities for elderly people, it could help restore these people's health, dignity, self-sufficiency, and perhaps even start a new vibrant phase of life for them.

Q. Ultrasound scans have shown that I have a fatty liver. My whole body is swollen, and I have several lumps in my breasts and thyroid. My blood cholesterol is very high, and I frequently throw up food. Could the liver flush help?

A. There is no medical therapy to date that can remove fat deposits from the liver. Nevertheless, you can prove to yourself and to your doctor that you can reduce and even eliminate all fatty deposits in the liver by clearing the liver's bile ducts of all gallstones. The liver may have accumulated these deposits for many reasons, including high protein, sugar, and alcohol consumption; stress; lack of proper sleep; and, foremost of all, to trap noxious substances. Whatever may be the original causes or causes of the congestion in your liver, if you repeatedly cleanse it, your liver will gradually improve and repair itself as much as possible. Consider taking another scan (although I do not generally recommend scans) after your sixth or eighth liver flush, and let your doctor compare it with the previous one. The difference will literally be like black and white. Once your liver is cleared of fatty deposits, similar deposits will also disappear from other parts of the body, such as breasts, thyroid, arteries, and so on. All of this, of course, is contingent upon your maintaining a balanced, low-protein, preferably vegan diet and a healthy lifestyle.

Q. Can taking Epsom salts have harmful side effects? I find that it causes soreness in my anus during the flush.

A. Epsom salts (magnesium sulfate) can be found in mountain regions and is contained in sea salts. It is also manufactured synthetically by combining natural minerals. So long as the liver is congested, Epsom salts have no harmful side effects. The soreness in your anus stems from the strong toxins that are being released during the liver flush, not from the Epsom salts. If your GI tract were completely clean of toxic waste material, the magnesium in the Epsom salts would simply be absorbed and cause no further bowel movements. (Magnesium is a powerful laxative.) There would be no irritation and, therefore, no side effects, such as cramps, gas, bad breath, and so forth. These forms of discomfort result only from the release of toxins. The Epsom salts undergo biochemical changes as they pass through your small intestine. In other words, Epsom salts that reach the colon no longer exist in the same form as when you ingested them.

If you find that, during a successful liver flush, the last eight to ten bowel movements in the morning or afternoon consist merely of water without any stones or white cholesterol components, you may reduce the dosage of the last two helpings of Epsom salts by one-half each. If you are totally intolerant of or allergic to Epsom salts, use magnesium citrate or try other natural colonic cleansers that work fast, such as castor oil, *colosan,* and *oxypowder.* The latter two products consist of a blend of various magnesium oxides. (See *Product Information* at the end of the book.) The disadvantage to most other colon cleansers is that, unlike Epsom salts, they do not open the bile ducts to release the gallstones into the intestinal tract nearly as well—an important aspect of the flush.

Q. Is any type of olive oil suitable for the liver flush?

A. The olive oil should be cold pressed and 100 percent pure. Usually olive oil that bears the label "Extra Virgin Olive Oil" is the best but, nevertheless, read the label carefully. It should state that the oil has not been mixed with other oils. Unfortunately, in some countries, olive oil is sold as "extra virgin" but contains 80 percent soy oil. Real olive oil has a greenish/golden color. Organic olive oil has the best taste. If you are not sure about its authenticity, test it by using the *kinesiology* muscle test.[37] Other oils have also been used, but may not be as effective as olive oil.

Q. I read on the Internet that the stones people passed during the liver flushes are just hardened lumps of olive oil. Is there any truth to this?

---

[37] There are many books and videotapes available that can teach you how to apply this simple testing method. Kinesiology muscle testing can tell you immediately whether a food product is suitable for you or not. There is also an exact description of the testing procedure in *Timeless Secrets of Health and Rejuvenation.*

A. There is an effort on behalf of certain well-known herbalists, doctors, and establishments to discredit the beneficial effects of the liver flush by stating that these gallstones are actually "soap stones" made of olive oil or are produced by the liver in response to the sudden ingestion of large quantities of olive oil. These individuals have their own reasons for making such statements, which is not for me to comment on. They have obviously never done a liver flush themselves. Otherwise they would realize what these stones are made of and what happens to their body when they release them. Below are a number of responses to such a claim:

1. Olive oil does not assume the putrid smell that emanates from most released gallstones. The smell is unlike that produced by fecal matter.

2. Olive oil cannot congeal into such relatively hard or dense structures, even if it were chemically altered and manipulated in a laboratory. This is even more impossible, given the short time frame the olive oil has to travel through the GI tract and the total unavailability of any thickening agents.

3. Analysis of released gallstones reveals that the majority contain all the basic ingredients that make up bile fluid. Organic matter may also be present. Many of these stones consist of layers and layers of old, dark-green bile, something that does not happen overnight. The rest of the stones are the typical calcified gallstones found in the gallbladder. The dark-red or black bilirubin stones some people pass during their flushes certainly cannot pass as olive oil "soap stones."

4. The olive oil mixture does not even go through the liver, as it would if it were combined with food. Therefore, during the liver flush, the liver does nothing but release gallstones and bile. Neither the liver nor the small intestine can act as a soap stone factory.

5. Once the liver and gallbladder are completely clean, no more gallstones are released after ingesting the oil/citrus juice mixture. If these stones were indeed made from olive oil, they would also occur during a liver flush done after the liver has been completely cleansed and all bile ducts are clear and open. However, this is not the case. The liver flush produces no more stones once the liver is clean, regardless how much olive oil one ingests. Besides, the olive oil consumed during liver flushes does not always produce the same results. During one flush only 50 stones may come out, whereas during the next one, as many as 1,000 may be expelled.

6. Because of intolerance to olive oil, some people have used, for example, clear-colored macadamia nut oil during their flushes and produced precisely the same green-colored stones. Cholesterol stones that exactly match these green stones can be found in the bile ducts of dissected livers.

7. If stones were just blobs of olive oil, why do so many people get cured from chronic illnesses such as asthma, allergies, cancer, heart disease, diabetes, and even paralysis, after passing numerous "soap stones" during their liver flushes?

8. Many people have released stones of different colors: black, red, green, white, yellow, and tan. Olive oil does not have coloring agents in it to produce stones of different colors.

9. People who have sent their stones in for chemical analysis have received reports that almost all the stones were made from cholesterol and salts. These constituents are identical to those in the cholesterol stones found in gallbladders that have been removed. A very small number of "stones" consisted of organic matter of unknown origin. These could easily have been trapped in the bile ducts along with the gallstones.

10. Quite a few individuals, including me myself, have sometimes passed green cholesterol stones on the evening of the flush, even before taking the olive oil mixture. Others, who had already done several liver flushes, have reported stones coming out during the apple juice phase, all without the help of olive oil. The stones that come out on their own have no different shape, color, and smell than the ones released during the actual flushes.

11. It is conventional medicine, and not the author, that proved the presence of cholesterol stones in the bile ducts of the liver. The medical term for these stones is "intrahepatic stones," or "biliary stones." These green stones, made of cholesterol and some bile constituents, are, in fact, oily and decompose when exposed to warmer air temperatures and oxygen. Cholesterol itself consists of about 96 percent water. These cholesterol stones are quickly broken down by destructive bacteria when released into the environment. This does not occur, however, while they are trapped in the bile ducts of the liver.

12. Plenty of photographs have been taken of dissected livers and are in the medical archives of university clinics that show the presence of these stones in the bile ducts of the liver.

13. It is a medically proven fact that millions of people regularly pass green sludge consisting of sometimes dozens of green cholesterol stones in response to eating a very fatty meal. These stones are **not** composed of the oils or fats that were ingested. They are forced out of the liver and gallbladder along with the expelled bile. Unfortunately, unlike during liver flushing, some of the stones get caught in the common bile duct or even in the pancreatic duct. There is no difference between the stones that are released involuntarily and those passed voluntarily during a liver flush.

The liver flush is not the result of a placebo effect. The calcified stones released by the gallbladder, usually after five to eight liver flushes, are identical to those found in dissected gallbladders. They do not disintegrate and remain stone hard. Only semicalcified stones may shrink in time; yet the calcified shell remains intact.

I personally suffered over forty gallbladder attacks during a period of more than ten years, and my gallbladder was packed with stones, causing a painful, short spinal scoliosis. Since my first liver flush I never suffered another attack. The scoliosis, among other health problems, vanished after my twelfth flush. After that, none of my yearly flushes has produced any stones, although I used exactly the same procedure. My gallbladder is completely clean and efficient now.

Thousands of people from all over the world have saved their gallbladders through liver flushing. Others have fully regained their health and even saved their own lives by doing this flush. Those who intentionally promote or spread the strange and unsubstantiated claim that liver flushing produces olive soap stones, rob their compatriots and themselves of the opportunity to take care of their own health. This is something they will have to live with.

Q. I am taking food supplements. Should I continue taking them while doing the liver flush?

A. It is best to avoid any supplements or medicines during the liver flush, unless they are essential. Besides, they are wasted as they are flushed out with the bile and Epsom salts. In addition, medicinal drugs and substances, such as sleeping pills, have a suppressive effect that can render the cleanse ineffective.

Q. I have done eight livers flushes so far and I feel great. Almost all of my symptoms, including stomach ulcers, sinusitis, and headaches, are gone without a trace. Altogether, I must have released about 2,500 stones. What I do not understand is why my first liver flush produced no stones whatsoever and the second one only six or seven small ones. During the following flush, I passed about a thousand, much to my amazement. Can you explain why I wasn't successful with the first two flushes?

A. You are one of those rare people whose major bile ducts in the liver were solidly congested with gallstones, and it took three flushes to soften the hardened structures and break them down. It is not true that the first two flushes were not successful. They were. They did the groundwork or "digging," and the following flushes just removed what was already dug up—thanks to your patience and persistence!

Q. During a total of five liver flushes, I have passed over 1,200 stones. My fifth flush, however, didn't release more than 20 stones. Does this mean that my liver is clean now?

A. Not necessarily. It may be that your five flushes have successfully removed all the stones that were held in one of the two major biliary duct networks, but the second one may still be blocked. Further cleansing will open it, too. You may even release more stones during future flushes than you did with the previous ones, since the most blocked and resistant bile ducts tend to open only once the lesser congested bile ducts have been opened up.

Q. Isn't it necessary after a liver flush to replenish electrolytes and intestinal flora?

A. Although it sounds reasonable to give back to the body what it has lost as part of the cleansing, I have found that it is far better to let the body take care of this. By doing so, the body is stimulated to take care of its own needs rather than forcing it to use eternally supplied "crutches." In addition, it is actually much easier to replenish electrolytes and friendly bacteria when the intestinal tract is clean. In fact, bacterial balance is usually restored within less than 48 hours.

Q. What role do gallstones play in children's diseases? You mention diabetes, but how about things like leukemia, juvenile rheumatoid arthritis, and so forth? Can a child have developed enough gallstones at a very young age to contribute to serious diseases?

A. It is becoming increasingly obvious that gallstones can form in children just as easily as they do in older people. In fact, age is not a risk factor at all for gallstones. Regardless of whether it is a child or an adult who regularly drinks diet sodas, eats hamburgers, or consumes low-fat foods, both of them will manufacture gallstones in direct response to such dietary choices. Many children are literally being poisoned by what they eat or drink, including the popular "healthy" breakfast cereals.[38] It is not surprising to find that many children today have already accumulated hundreds, and sometimes thousands, of gallstones in their liver. The more they have gathered, the more likely they are to suffer from such serious illnesses as the ones you have mentioned. I developed gallstones before the age of 6 and began to experience debilitating illnesses from age 8, just from eating foods rich in animal protein. Children age 10 or older can do liver flushes; however, they should use only half the dosage of all the ingredients, that is, apple juice, olive oil, Epsom salts, and juice. Children aged 16 or older can use the adult dosage, unless their body frame is still very small.

Q. How long does it take for an average, pea-sized gallstone to form in the liver? Is it possible to form them as fast as you can cleanse them?

A. This depends on how many gallstones you have already accumulated, what kind of foods or beverages you consume, your emotional state, and your lifestyle. Alcohol, coffee, other stimulants, and diuretics, such as sugar and meat, can quickly

---

[38] To learn more about the astounding scientific research conducted on breakfast cereals, see *Timeless Secrets of Health and Rejuvenation.*

congeal bile and, thereby, form stones. Some stones can reach pea-size within several weeks. Therefore, to attain and then maintain a clean liver, I recommend applying the dietary and lifestyle changes I have noted in this book, in addition to carrying out the liver flushes.

Q. I have a lot of moles on my arms and forearms, some that have developed within the last year. Is this an indication of gallstones, the same as liver spots on the back of the hands, or brown patches on the temple area? Do moles and skin discolorations disappear as the liver is cleansed of gallstones?

A. Most of these skin blemishes appear in direct relation to existing or newly developing gallstones in the bile ducts of the liver and gallbladder. Many of them tend to fade and disappear once the liver and gallbladder are completely clean or, in some cases, after releasing most of the gallstones. Another cause of moles, freckles, and liver spots is a deficiency in ionic selenium (see *Take Ionic Essential Minerals* in Chapter 5). To remove moles through external applications, see my book *Timeless Secrets of Health and Rejuvenation.*

Q. How many colonics does a person generally need to do to be clean?

A. The number of colon treatments required varies with the individual and his or her prevailing condition, diet, and lifestyle. In some cases, the waste is so hard and affixed to the colon wall that it may take a series of up to seven colonics to sufficiently soften and loosen this *accumulated fecal material.* Some people may not have startling results for the first few treatments. That is why a series of at least three treatments, once per week, is recommended and advisable for anyone who has never done any colon cleansing. It is also important that you monitor your colon health by listening to any pain signals or stiffness that may occur in the neck, shoulders, low back, pelvic area, or arms. These aches and pains will let you know that it is time again for another colon cleanse. To detect any hidden areas of pain or tension in the colon, you may gently press the abdominal area about 2 to 4 inches away from the navel—on the left of it, above it, and on the right of it. Check for any tender spots or hardness.

Q. Do colonics have harmful side effects?
A. Colonics have no known harmful side effects. It is possible, however, for some people to have cold-like symptoms or a headache after a colonic. The cause is toxins that have been lying dormant in the colon and are now being flushed out. Some waste deposits, though, may only be partially removed not be cleared out, and a small amount may be reabsorbed into the body. Such a healing crisis generally passes quickly, and the person will realize a greater feeling of well-being with further treatments. Having dealt with colonic irrigation for nearly two decades, I have not yet seen any ill effects.

Q. Can colonics damage normal intestinal flora?

A. The normal intestinal flora, consisting of friendly bacteria, will not be disturbed. The first half of the colon is responsible for generating and gathering the *intestinal flora* required for balanced colon functions. The appendix serves as the main breeding place for beneficial bacteria. When food is not digested properly, feces tend to attach to the inside of the bowel. Layer upon layer of fecal encrustation inhibits the lining of the intestine from producing the necessary *intestinal flora*. This also leads to poor lubrication of the intestinal lining and intensifies the congestion and generates *toxemia*. This, in turn, upsets the normal *acid-alkaline balance* (pH) and further inhibits the growth of beneficial bacteria. Consequently, this imbalance invites destructive bacteria to overpopulate the gut. (Destructive bacteria help to break down waste, but produce strong toxins as a result of this action.) Colon cleansing helps to restore the normal pH-value in the bowel. In this more supportive environment, the *beneficial bacteria* will once again thrive, and disease-causing bacteria will find it more difficult to develop.

Concluding Remarks

Cleansing the liver is not something that was invented recently. All ancient cultures and civilizations knew of the necessity to keep the liver clean. Plenty of useful cleansing formulas still exist that were handed down through the generations, either by ancestral education or by traditional healers. Although the exact mechanisms of these time-tested cleansing procedures were not as well understood then as they are today (through methods of scientific understanding and investigation), they are no less valid, scientific, and effective than any newly proven therapy. Medical science has yet to come to terms with the fact that numerous useful methods of healing have worked for millions of people throughout the ages and can make all the difference in the treatment of the most threatening diseases that plague modern societies.

Every house and appliance requires some form of maintenance or repair work from time to time; otherwise, it will lose its ability to carry out the true purpose for which it was designed. The same principle applies to the liver. No other organ in the body besides the brain is as complex and has as many vital functions as the liver. We clean our teeth and wash our skin every day because we know that exposure to food, air, chemicals, and normal metabolic processes tends to leave residues that can make us feel unclean and uncomfortable. Not many people, however, think that the same principle of cleaning also applies to the inner parts of the body. The lungs, skin, intestines, kidneys, and liver deal with a tremendous amount of internally produced waste, which is a necessary by-product of breathing, digestion, and metabolism.

Under normal circumstances, the body can properly deal with the metabolic waste products that accumulate daily by eliminating them safely from the system. These normal circumstances include eating nutritious and organic foods, living in a pollution-free environment, having plenty of physical movement and exercise, and living a balanced, joyful lifestyle. Yet how many of us can claim to live such fulfilling lives? What happens when our diet, lifestyle, and environment are no longer balanced enough to suit the body's requirements for energy, nourishment, and flawless circulation? One of the organs that suffers the most from an overload of toxic chemicals, poor quality of food, and lack of exercise is the liver. Hence, it is of utmost importance for everyone who is concerned about their health to ensure that their liver is cleansed and remains free of any obstructions.

Cleansing the liver is not something someone else can do for you. Rather, it is a self-help method that requires a profound sense of self-responsibility and trust in the natural, innate wisdom of the body. You will only feel drawn toward liver flushing when you know deep within yourself that this is something you absolutely have to do. If you do not feel this way, it may be best to put this book aside for the time being and wait. When the time is right, you will feel the definite impulse or desire to improve your liver's functioning.

Although the liver flush is not a cure for diseases, it sets the precondition for the body to heal itself. In fact, it is rare for an ailment not to improve by increasing liver performance. To understand the great significance of the liver flush, one needs to personally experience how it feels to have a liver that has been relieved of two handfuls of gallstones. For many people, the liver flush has been an "amazing" experience—reason enough for me to share it with those willing to help themselves.

Product Information

To order books, *Ener-chi Art* pictures, and Ionized Stones
please contact:

Ener-Chi Wellness Center, LLC

Web site: www.ener-chi.com
Toll free: 1-866-258-4006 (USA)
Local (709) 570-7401 (Canada)

See Suppliers List below for products mentioned in this book.

To obtain a complete list of suppliers
and to order other health-promoting products
recommended by the author,
please visit:

Web site: www.ener-chi.com

Suppliers List

All address are in the United States, unless otherwise specified.

Ionic Water-Soluble Minerals

Eniva Corporation
P.O. Box 49755
Minneapolis, MN 55449

Toll-free: 1-866-999-9191
Tel: 763-398-0005
Fax: 763-795-8890
Web site: www.eniva.com

Note: To order any products from Eniva, you require a sponsor name and ID. You may use the name and ID of the author, Andreas Moritz, #13462.

Kornax Enterprises, LLS (for the WaterOZ products)
P.O. Box 783
Lyons, CO 80540

Toll-free:1-877-328-1744 (U.S. & Canada)
Tel: 303-823-5813
Fax: 303-823-6780
Web site: www.kornax.com

Unrefined Sea Salt

Redmond Minerals, Inc.
P.O. Box 219
Redmond, UT 84652
Toll-free: 1-800-367-7258
Tel: 435-529-7402
Fax: 435-529-7486
mail@redmondminerals.com
www.realsalt.com

Grain and Salt Society
273 Fairway Dr.
Asheville, NC 28805
Toll-free: 1-800-TOP-SALT (1-800-867-7258)
Fax: 1-828-299-1640
topsalt@aol.com
www.celtic-seasalt.com

Colema Board, Colon Cleanse Equipments

Colema Boards of California, Inc.
3660 Main St., Suite C
Cottonwood, CA 96022
Tel: 1-800-745-2446
http://www.colema.com/

Home and Professional Colon Hydrotherapy Equipment

www.homecolonics.com/

thecolonet.com

Herbs for the Kidney Cleanse and Liver Tea

**The Present Moment
Books & Herbs**
3546 Grand Avenue
Minneapolis, MN 55409

Note: Herbs are very fresh and
potent and come already mixed.

Mail Order: 1-800-378-3245
 612-824-3157
Fax: 612-824-2031
herbshop@presentmoment.com
www.presentmoment.com

Clay Bath Kits
(to remove heavy metals)

www.magneticclay.com
www.magneticclaybaths.com, 800-257-3315

Products for Alternative Versions of the Liver Cleanse

- **Gold Coin Grass**
- **Chinese Gentian and Bupleurum**

Prime Health Products
15 Belfield Rd., Unit C
Toronto, Ontario, Canada M9W
Tel: 416-248-2930, 416-248-0415
E-mail:
jchang@sensiblehealth.com
Fax: 416-248-0415, 1-416-233-5347
Web site: sensiblehealth.com

- **Chanca Piedra Extract**

Ashaninka
www.ashaninka.com

- **Malic Acid Powder, Food Grade**

Presque Isle Wine Cellars
94440 W Main Rd.
North East, PA 16428
Tel: 1-814-725-1314
Web site: www.piwine.com

- **Colosan**

Family Health News
9845 N.E 2nd Ave.
Miami Shores, FL 33138
Tel: 1-800-284-6263
305-759-9500
Web site:
www.familyhealthnews.com

Water Treatment

- **Water Ionizers**

Fern's Nutrition
16932 Gothard, Suite H
Huntington Beach, CA 92647
Tel: 714-841-5349
fernshealth@fernsnutrition.com
www.fernsnutrition.com

- **H2O Concepts International**

6000 S. Eastern, Suite #4D
Las Vegas, NV 89119
Toll-free: 1-888-275-4261
Tel: 702-270-9697
www.h2oconcepts.com/

• Puritec (Whole house)	• Prill Water
Toll Free: 1-888-491-4100 Local: 702-562-8802 www.puritec.com	Global Light Network http://www.Global-Light-Network.com

Botanical Names for Kidney Cleanse Herbs

Marjoram	Origanum majorana
Cat's claw	Uncaria tomentosa
Comfrey root	Symphytum officinale
Fennel seed	Foeniculum vulgare
Chicory herb	Chichorium intybus
Uva ursi or bearberry	Arctostaphylos
Hydrangea root	Hydrangea arborescens
Gravel root	Eupatorium purpureum
Marshmallow root	Althaea officinalis
Golden rod herb	Solidago virgaurea

Botanical Names for Liver Herbs

Dandelion root	Taraxacum officinale
Comfrey root	Symphytum officinale
Licorice root	Glycyrrhiza glabra
Agrimony	Agrimonia eupatoria
Wild yam root	Dioscorea villosa
Barberry bark	Berberis vulgaris
Bearsfoot	Polymnia uvedalia
Tanners oak bark	Quercus robur
Milk thistle herb	Silybum marianum

ABOUT THE AUTHOR

Andreas Moritz is a medical intuitive; a practitioner of Ayurveda, iridology, shiatsu, and vibrational medicine; a writer; and an artist. Born in southwest Germany in 1954, Moritz had to deal with several severe illnesses from an early age, which compelled him to study diet, nutrition, and various methods of natural healing while still a child.

By the age of 20, he had completed his training in both iridology—the diagnostic science of eye interpretation—and dietetics. In 1981, he began studying Ayurvedic medicine in India and finished his training as a qualified practitioner of Ayurveda in New Zealand in 1991. Rather than being satisfied with merely treating the symptoms of illness, Moritz has dedicated his life's work to understanding and treating the root causes of illness. Because of this holistic approach, he has had great success with cases of terminal disease where conventional methods of healing proved futile.

Since 1988, he has practiced the Japanese healing art of shiatsu, which has given him insights into the energy system of the body. In addition, he devoted eight years of research into consciousness and its important role in the field of mind/body medicine.

Andreas Moritz is the author of *Timeless Secrets of Health and Rejuvenation, Lifting the Veil of Duality, Cancer Is Not a Disease, It's Time to Come Alive, Heart Disease No More, Simple Steps to Total Health, Diabetes—No More, Ending the AIDS Myth* and *Heal Yourself with Sunlight.*

During his extensive travels throughout the world, he has consulted with heads of state and members of government in Europe, Asia, and Africa, and has lectured widely on the subjects of health, mind/body medicine, and spirituality. His popular *Timeless Secrets of Health and Rejuvenation* workshops assist people in taking responsibility for their own health and well-being. Moritz has a free forum, "Ask Andreas Moritz," on the large health website curezone.com (five million readers and increasing). Although he recently stopped writing for the forum, it contains an extensive archive of his answers to thousands of questions on a variety of health topics.

Since taking up residence in the United States in 1998, Moritz has been involved in developing a new and innovative system of healing—called *Ener-Chi Art*—that targets the root causes of many chronic illnesses. Ener-Chi Art consists of a series of light ray–encoded oil paintings that can instantly restore vital energy flow (Chi) in the organs and systems of the body. Moritz is also the founder of *Sacred Santémony—Divine Chanting for Every Occasion,* a powerful system of specially generated frequencies of sound that can transform deep-seated fears, allergies, traumas, and mental or emotional blocks into useful opportunities for growth and inspiration within a matter of moments.

Other Books, Products, and Services
by the Author

Timeless Secrets of Health and Rejuvenation –
Breakthrough Medicine for the 21st Century (488 pages)

This book meets the increasing demand for a clear and comprehensive guide that can help make people self-sufficient regarding their health and well-being. It answers some of the most pressing questions of our time: How does illness arise? Who heals, who doesn't? Are we destined to be sick? What causes aging? Is it reversible? What are the major causes of disease, and how can we eliminate them?

Topics include: The placebo and the mind/body mystery; the laws of illness and health; the four most common risk factors for disease; digestive disorders and their effects on the rest of the body; the wonders of our biological rhythms and how to restore them if disrupted; how to create a life of balance; why to choose a vegetarian diet; cleansing the liver, gallbladder, kidneys, and colon; removing allergies; giving up smoking naturally; using sunlight as medicine; the "new" causes of heart disease, cancer, diabetes, and AIDS; and antibiotics, blood transfusions, ultrasound scans, and immunization programs under scrutiny.

Timeless Secrets of Health and Rejuvenation sheds light on all major issues of health care and reveals that most medical treatments, including surgery, blood transfusions, and pharmaceutical drugs are avoidable when certain key functions in the body are restored through the natural methods described in the book. The reader also learns about the potential dangers of medical diagnosis and treatment, as well as the reasons vitamin supplements, "health foods," low-fat products, "wholesome" breakfast cereals, diet foods, and diet programs may have contributed to the current health crisis rather than helped to resolve it. The book includes a complete program of health care, which is primarily based on the ancient medical system of Ayurveda and the vast amount of experience Andreas Moritz has gained in the field of health restoration during the past thirty years.

Lifting the Veil of Duality –
Your Guide to Living without Judgment

"Do you know that there is a place inside you -- hidden beneath the appearance of thoughts, feelings, and emotions – that does not know the difference between good and evil, right and wrong, light and dark? From that place you embrace the opposite values of life as *One*. In this sacred place you are at peace with yourself and at peace with your world." *Andreas Moritz*

In *Lifting the Veil of Duality,* Andreas Moritz poignantly exposes the illusion of duality. He outlines a simple way to remove every limitation that you have imposed upon yourself during the course of living duality. You will be prompted to see yourself and the world through a new lens – the lens of clarity, discernment, and non-judgment. You will also discover that mistakes, accidents, coincidences, negativity, deception, injustice, wars, crime, and terrorism all have a deeper purpose and meaning in the larger scheme of things. So naturally, much of what you will read may conflict with the beliefs you currently hold. Yet you are not asked to change your beliefs or opinions. Instead, you are asked to have *an open mind,* for only an open mind can enjoy freedom from judgment.

Our personal views and worldviews are currently challenged by a crisis of identity. Some are being shattered altogether. The collapse of our current World Order, forces humanity to deal with the most basic issues of existence. You can no longer avoid taking responsibility for the things that happen to you. When you *do* accept responsibility, you also empower and heal yourself.

Lifting the Veil of Duality shows you how you create or subdue your ability to fulfill your desires. Furthermore, you will find intriguing explanations about the mystery of time, the truth and illusion of reincarnation, the oftentimes misunderstood value of prayer, what makes relationships work, and why so often they don't. Find out why injustice is an illusion that has managed to haunt us throughout the ages. Learn about our original separation from the Source of life and what this means with regard to the current waves of instability and fear so many of us are experiencing.

Discover how to identify the angels living amongst us and why we all have light-bodies. You will have the opportunity to find the ultimate God within you and discover why a God seen as separate from yourself keeps you from being in your Divine Power and happiness. In addition, you can find out how to heal yourself at a moment's notice. Read all about the "New Medicine" and the destiny of the old medicine, the old economy, the old religion, and the old world.

It's Time to Come Alive!
Start Using the Amazing Healing Powers of Your Body, Mind, and Spirit Today!

In this book, the author brings to light man's deep inner need for spiritual wisdom in life and helps the reader develop a new sense of reality that is based on love, power, and compassion. He describes our relationship with the natural world in detail and discusses how we can harness its tremendous powers for our personal and humanity's benefit. *Time to Come Alive* challenges some of our most commonly held beliefs and offers a way out of the emotional restrictions and physical limitations we have created in our lives.

Topics include: What shapes our destiny; using the power of intention; secrets of defying the aging process; doubting - the cause of failure; opening the heart; material wealth and spiritual wealth; fatigue – the major cause of stress; methods of emotional transformation; techniques of primordial healing; how to increase the health of the five senses; developing spiritual wisdom; the major causes of today's earth changes; entry into the new world; twelve gateways to heaven on earth; and many more.

Cancer is Not a Disease!
It's A Survival Mechanism
Discover Cancer's Hidden Purpose, Heal its Root Causes, and be Healthier Than Ever!

In *Cancer is Not a Disease,* Andreas Moritz proves the point that cancer is the physical symptom that reflects our body's final attempt to deal with life-threatening cell congestion and toxins. He claims that removing the underlying conditions that force the body to produce cancerous cells, sets the preconditions for complete healing of our body, mind, and emotions.

This book confronts you with a radically new understanding of cancer – one that revolutionized the current cancer model. On the average, today's conventional "treatments" of killing, cutting out, or burning cancerous cells offer most patients a remission rate of a mere 7%, and the majority of these survivors are "cured" for just five years or fewer. Prominent cancer researcher and professor at the University of California at Berkeley, Dr. Hardin Jones, stated: "Patients are as well, or better off, untreated..." Any published success figures in cancer survival statistics are offset by equal or better scores among those receiving no treatment at all. More people are killed by cancer treatments than are saved by them.

Cancer is Not a Disease shows you why traditional cancer treatments are often fatal, what actually causes cancer, and how you can remove the obstacles that prevent the body from healing itself. Cancer is not an attempt on your life; on the contrary, this "dread disease" is the body's final, desperate effort to save your life. Unless we change our perception of what cancer really is, it will continue to threaten the life of nearly one out of every two people. This book opens a door for those who wish to turn feelings of victimhood into empowerment and self-mastery, and disease into health.

Topics of the book include:

- Reasons the body is forced to develop cancer cells
- How to identify and remove the causes of cancer
- Why most cancers disappear by themselves, without medical intervention
- Why radiation, chemotherapy, and surgery never cure cancer
- Why some people survive cancer despite undergoing dangerously radical treatments
- The roles of fear, frustration, low self-worth, and repressed anger in the origination of cancer
- How to turn self-destructive emotions into energies that

promote health and vitality
- Spiritual lessons behind cancer

Heart Disease No More!
Make Peace with Your Heart and Heal Yourself
(Excerpted from Timeless Secrets of Health & Rejuvenation)

Less than one hundred years ago, heart disease was an extremely rare disease. Today it kills more people in the developed world than all other causes of death combined. Despite the vast amount of financial resources spent on finding a cure for heart disease, the current medical approaches remain mainly symptom-oriented and do not address the underlying causes.

Even worse: There is overwhelming evidence to show that the treatment of heart disease or its presumed precursors, such as high blood pressure, hardening of the arteries and high cholesterol, does not only prevent a real cure but can easily lead to chronic heart failure. The patient's heart may still beat, but not strong enough to feel vital and alive.

Without removing the underlying causes of heart disease and its precursors, there is little, if any, protection against it. Heart attacks can strike regardless whether you have had a coronary bypass done or stents placed inside your arteries. According to research, these procedures fail to prevent heart attacks or reduce mortality rates.

Heart Disease No More, excerpted from the author's bestselling book, Timeless Secrets of Health & Rejuvenation, puts the responsibility for healing where it belongs, that is, to the heart, mind and body of each individual. It provides you with the practical insights about how heart disease develops, what causes it and what you can do to prevent and reverse it for good, regardless of a possible genetic predisposition.

Diabetes - No More!
Discover and Heal Its True Causes
(Excerpted from Timeless Secrets of Health & Rejuvenation)

According to this bestselling author, diabetes is not a disease; in the vast majority of cases, it is a complex mechanism of protection or survival that the body chooses to avoid the possibly fatal consequences of an unhealthful diet and lifestyle.

Despite the body's ceaseless self-preservation efforts (which we call diseases), millions of people suffer or die unnecessarily from such consequences. The imbalanced blood sugar level in diabetes is but a symptom of illness, not the illness itself. By developing diabetes, the body is neither doing something wrong nor is it trying to commit suicide. The current diabetes epidemic is man-made, or rather, factory-made, and, therefore, can be halted and reversed through simple but effective changes in diet and lifestyle. *Diabetes - No More* provides you with essential information on the various causes of diabetes and how anyone can avoid them.

To stop the diabetes epidemic we need to create the right circumstances that allow the body to heal. Just as there is a mechanism to become diabetic, there is also a mechanism to reverse it. Find out how!

This book was excerpted from the bestselling book, Timeless Secrets of Health and Rejuvenation.

Ending The AIDS Myth
It's Time To Heal The TRUE Causes!
(Excerpted from Timeless Secrets of Health and Rejuvenation)

Contrary to common belief, there is no scientific evidence to this day that AIDS is a contagious disease. The current AIDS theory falls short in predicting the kind of AIDS disease an infected person may be manifesting, and there is no accurate system to determine how long it will take for the disease to develop. In addition, the current HIV/AIDS theory contains no reliable information that can help identify those who are at risk of developing AIDS.

On the other hand, published research actually proves that HIV only extremely rarely spreads heterosexually and cannot be responsible for an epidemic that involves millions of AIDS victims around the world. Furthermore, it is an established fact that the retrovirus HIV, which is composed of human gene fragments, is incapable of destroying human cells. However, cell destruction is the main characteristic of every AIDS disease.

Even the principal discoverer of HIV, Luc Montagnier, no longer believes that HIV is solely responsible for causing AIDS. In fact, he showed that HIV alone could not cause AIDS. There is increasing evidence that AIDS may be a toxicity syndrome or metabolic disorder that is caused by immunity risk factors, including heroin, sex drugs, antibiotics, commonly prescribed AIDS drugs, rectal intercourse, starvation, malnutrition and dehydration.

Dozens of prominent scientists working at the forefront of the AIDS research are now openly questioning the virus hypothesis of AIDS. Find out why! *Ending the AIDS Myth* also shows you what really causes the shutdown of the immune system and what needs to be done to avoid it!

Heal Yourself with Sunlight (March 2007)
Use Its Secret Medicinal Powers to Help Cure Cancer, Heart Disease, Hypertension, Diabetes, Arthritis, Infectious Diseases, and much more.
(Excerpted from Timeless Secrets of Health & Rejuvenation)

Hear the Whispers, Live Your Dream (July 2007)
A Fanfare of Inspiration

All books are available as paperback copies and electronic books through the Ener-Chi Wellness Center

Website: http://www.ener-chi.com
Email: andmor@ener-chi.com
Toll free (1-866) 258-4006 (USA)
Local (709) 570-7401 (Canada)

Sacred Santémony – for Emotional Healing

Sacred Santémony is a unique healing system that uses sounds from specific words to balance deep emotional/spiritual imbalances. The powerful words produced in Sacred Santémony are made from whole-brain use of the letters of the *ancient language* – a language that is comprised of the basic sounds that underlie and bring forth all physical manifestation. The letters of the ancient language vibrate at a much higher level than our modern languages, and when combined to form whole words, they generate feelings of peace and harmony (Santémony) to calm the storms of unrest, violence, and turmoil, both internal and external.

In April, 2002 I spontaneously began to chant sounds that are meant to improve certain health conditions. These sounds resembled chants by Native Americans, Tibetan monks, Vedic pundits (Sanskrit), and languages from other star systems (not known on planet Earth). Within two weeks, I was able to bring forth sounds that would instantly remove emotional blocks and resistance or aversion to certain situations and people, foods, chemicals, thought forms, beliefs, etc. The following are but a few examples of what Sacred Santémony is able to assist you with:

⇒ Reducing or removing fear that is related to death, disease, the body, foods, harmful chemicals, parents and other people, lack of abundance, impoverishment, phobias, environmental threats, the future and the past, unstable economic trends, political unrest, etc.

⇒ Clearing or reducing a recent or current hurt, disappointment, or anger resulting from past emotional trauma or negative experiences in life.

⇒ Cleansing of the *Akashic Records* (a recording of all experiences the soul has gathered throughout all life streams) from persistent fearful elements, including the idea and concept that we are separate from and not one with Spirit, God, or our Higher Self.

⇒ Setting the preconditions for you to resolve your karmic issues, not through pain and suffering, but through creativity and joy.

⇒ Improving or clearing up allergies and intolerances to foods, chemical substances, pesticides, herbicides, air pollutants, radiation, medical drugs, pharmaceutical byproducts, etc.

⇒ Undoing the psycho-emotional root causes of any chronic illness, including cancer, heart disease, MS, diabetes, arthritis, brain disorders, depression, etc.

⇒ Resolving other difficulties or barriers in life by "converting" them into the useful blessings that they really are.

To arrange for a personal Sacred Santémony session with Andreas Moritz, please follow the same directions as given for telephone consultations.

Ener-Chi Art

Andreas Moritz has developed a new system of healing and rejuvenation designed to restore the basic life energy (Chi) of an organ or a system in the body within a matter of seconds. Simultaneously, it also helps balance the emotional causes of illness.

Eastern approaches to healing, such as acupuncture and Shiatsu, are intended to enhance well-being by stimulating and balancing the flow of Chi to the various organs and systems of the body. In a similar manner, the energetics of Ener-Chi Art is designed to restore a balanced flow of Chi throughout the body.

According to most ancient systems of health and healing, the balanced flow of Chi is the key determinant for a healthy body and mind. When Chi flows through the body unhindered, health and vitality are maintained. By contrast, if the flow of Chi is disrupted or reduced, health and vitality tend to decline.

A person can determine the degree to which the flow of Chi is balanced in the body's organs and systems by using a simple muscle testing procedure. To reveal the effectiveness of Ener-Chi Art, it is important to apply this test both before and after viewing each Ener-Chi Art picture.

To allow for easy application of this system, Andreas has created a number of healing paintings that have been "activated" through a unique procedure that imbues each work of art with specific color rays (derived from the higher dimensions). To receive the full benefit of an Ener-Chi Art picture, all that is necessary is to look at it for less than a minute. During this time, the flow of Chi within the organ or system becomes fully restored.

When applied to all the organs and systems of the body, Ener-Chi Art sets the precondition for the whole body to heal and rejuvenate itself.

Ener-Chi Ionized Stones

Ener-Chi Ionized Stones are stones and crystals that have been energized, activated, and imbued with life force through a special process introduced by Andreas Moritz, the founder of Ener-Chi Art.

Stone ionization has not been attempted before because stones and rocks have rarely been considered useful in the field of healing. Yet, stones have the inherent power to hold and release vast amounts of information and energy. Once ionized, they exert a balancing influence on everything with which they come into contact. The ionization of stones may be one of our keys to survival in a world that is experiencing high-level pollution and destruction of its eco-balancing systems.

In the early evolutionary stages of Earth, every particle of matter within the mantle of the planet, contained within it the blueprint of the entire planet, just as every cell of our body contains within its DNA structure, the blueprint of our entire body. The blueprint information within every particle of matter is still there – it has simply fallen into a dormant state. The ionization process "reawakens" this original blueprint information and enables the associated energies to be released. In this sense, Ener-Chi Ionized Stones are alive and conscious, and are able to energize, purify, and balance any natural substance with which they come into contact.

Potential Uses for Ionized Stones

Drinking Ionized Water
Placing an Ionized Stone next to a glass of water for about half a minute ionizes the water. Ionized water is a powerful cleanser that aids digestion and metabolism, and energizes the entire body.

Eating Ionized Foods

Placing an Ionized Stone next to your food for about half a minute ionizes and balances it. Due to the pollution particles in our atmosphere and soil, even natural organic foods are usually somewhat polluted. Such foods are also impacted by ozone depletion and exposure to electro-magnetic radiation in our planetary environment. These negative effects tend to be neutralized through the specified use of Ionized Stones.

Ionized Foot Bath

By placing Ionized Stones (preferably pebbles with rounded surfaces) under the soles of the feet, while the feet are immersed in water, the body begins to break down toxins and waste materials into harmless organic substances.

Enhancing Healing Therapies

Ionized Stones are ideal for enhancing the effects of any healing therapy. For example, "LaStone Therapy" is a popular new therapy that is offered in some innovative health spas. This involves placing warm stones on key energy points of the body. If these stones were ionized prior to being placed on the body, the healing effects would be enhanced. In fact, placing Ionized Stones on any weak or painful part of the body, including the corresponding chakra, has healthful benefits. If crystals play a role in the therapy, ionizing them first greatly amplifies their positive effects.

Aura and Chakra Balancing

Holding an Ionized Stone or Ionized Crystal in the middle section of the spinal column for about one-half minute balances all of the chakras, or energy centers, and tends to keep them in balance for several weeks or even months. Since energy imbalances in the chakras and auric field are one of the major causes of health problems, this balancing procedure is a powerful way to enhance health and well-being.

Attach to Main Water Pipe in Your Home

Attaching a stone to the main water pipe will ionize your water and make it more absorbable and energized.

Place in or near the Electrical Fuse Box in Your Home

By placing a larger Ionized Stone in, above, or below the fuse box in your house, the harmful effects of electromagnetic radiation become nullified. You can verify this by doing the muscle test (as shown on the instruction sheet for Ener-Chi Art) in front of a TV or computer, both before and after placing the stone on the fuse box. If you don't have a fuse box that is readily accessible, you can place a stone next to the electrical cable of your appliances or near their power sockets.

Use in Conjunction with Ener-Chi Art

Ionized Stones may be used to enhance the effects of Ener-Chi Art pictures. Simply place an Ionized Stone over the related area of the body while viewing an Ener-Chi Art picture. For example, if you are viewing the Ener-Chi Art picture related to the heart, hold an ionized stone over the heart area while viewing the picture. The nature of the energies involved in the pictures and the stones is similar. Accordingly, if the stones are used in combination with the pictures, a resonance is created which greatly enhances the overall effect.

Creating an Enhanced Environment

Placing an Ionized Stone near the various items that surround you for about half a minute helps to create a more energized and balanced environment. The Ionized Stones affect virtually all natural materials, such as wood floors, wood or metal furniture, stone walls, and brick or stone fireplaces. In work areas, especially near computers, it is a good idea to place one or more Ionized Stones in strategic locations. The same applies to sleeping areas, such as putting stones under your bed or pillow.

Improving Plant Growth

Placing Ionized Stones next to a plant or flowerpot may increase their health and beauty. This automatically ionizes the water they receive, whether they are indoor or outdoor plants. The same applies to vegetable plants and organic gardens.

Creating More Ionized Stones

Make any number of ionized stones by simply holding your "seed stone" against any other stones or crystals for 40-50 seconds. Your new stones will have the same effects as the seed stone.

Telephone Consultations

For a Personal Telephone Consultation with Andreas Moritz, please:

1. Call or send an email with your name, phone number, address, digital picture (if you have one) of your face and any other relevant information to:

E-mail: andmor@ener-chi.com

Telephone: 1 (864) 895-6285 (USA)

2. Set up an appointment for the length of time you choose to spend with him. A comprehensive consultation lasts two hours or more. Shorter consultations deal with all the questions you may have and any information that is relevant to your specific health issue(s).

For current fees please visit the consultation page at:
http://www.ener-chi.com

To order Books, Ener-chi Art pictures and Ionized Stones please contact:

Ener-Chi Wellness Center, LLC

Web Site: http://www.ener-chi.com
Toll free: 1(866) 258-4006 (USA)
Local (709) 570-7401 (Canada)

INDEX

216

Hernia, 4, 42
Herpes, 8
Hodgkin's disease, 42
Homeostasis, 2, 3, 25, 159, 161
Horizontal wrinkles across the bridge
of the nose, 65
Hormonal imbalances, 4
Hormonal Imbalances, 36
Hormones, 1, 2, 13, 15, 31, 42, 43, 51,
55, 56, 90, 99, 100, 101, 102, 103,
104, 142, 147, 148, 149, 151, 164,
167
Hypersensitivity, 18
see also allergies, 18
to drugs, alcohol, aspirin, fungi,
food additives, etc, 18
Hypertension, 28, 52, 66, 96
hypo-parathyroidism, 43
Hypothyroidism, 97, 98, 173

I

Immune cells, 57, 149
Immune system, 9, 17, 24, 34, 37, 38,
44, 55, 56, 57, 58, 60, 91, 100, 127,
141, 147, 148, 150, 153, 155, 159,
163, 205
*most of it is located in the intestinal
wall*, 56
Immunoglobulins, 57
Impotence, 4, 60
Inadequately digested foods, 24
Infarction, 30, 52
Infection, xvi, 2, 8, 12, 13, 16, 22, 23,
37, 38, 48, 60, 108, 119, 120, 122,
147, 159, 163, 171
inferior vena cava, 27, 37
Infertility, 60, 97, 101
Inner and Outer Beauty, viii, 166
Insomnia, 5, 98, 101
Insulin, 13, 43, 132
& diabetes, 44
Intestinal Diseases, v, 22
Intestinal juice, 8, 22, 23
Intestine large, xvi, 10, 22, 24, 36, 53,
69, 70, 108, 120, 126, 127, 129, 179
its size, 22
Intestine small, 5, 8, 10, 13, 19, 22, 23,
31, 38, 44, 54, 65, 68, 78, 82, 105,
108, 130, 183, 184
its size, 22

Intestines, xviii, 5, 6, 8, 9, 10, 11, 23,
24, 32, 36, 39, 52, 54, 59, 65, 69,
79, 81, 82, 92, 108, 130, 131, 163,
167, 178, 191
intrahepatic stones, xviii, 76, 185
Intrahepatic stones, xviii, 76, 185
Ionic Minerals, 51, 129
Ionized Stones, 146, 193, 208, 209,
210, 211, 212
Ionized Water, viii, 134, 209
irritable bowel syndrome, 42, 78, 129
Ischemia, 52

J

Jaundice, 13, 18
Joint diseases, 5
Joints, v, 42, 48, 56, 57, 58, 59, 88,
163, 164, 174
most susceptible to disease, 56
types of joints, 56

K

Kapha body types, 144
Kidney, vii, xvi, 5, 16, 33, 42, 48, 49,
50, 59, 62, 66, 72, 88, 96, 104, 107,
120, 130, 131, 132, 133, 134, 137,
148, 153, 194, 196
infection, xvi
Kidney stones, 48
*symptoms indicating kidney
malfunction*, 49
Uric acid stones, 48
when filtration is disrupted, 47
Kidney Cleanse, vii, 50, 59, 120, 132,
148
*additional measures to take with
large stones*, 134
herbs (Ingredients), 133
Kidney diseases, 5
Kidney failure, xvi, 33, 48
Kidney infection, 48
Knee problems, 5
Kupffer cells, 2

L

Lancet, 28, 95, 107
Laproscopy, 107
Large intestine, xvi, 10, 22, 24, 36, 53,
69, 70, 108, 120, 126, 127, 129, 179

NOTES